AS LEVEL

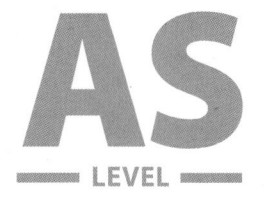

LIFE & HEALTH SCIENCES
FOR CCEA AS LEVEL

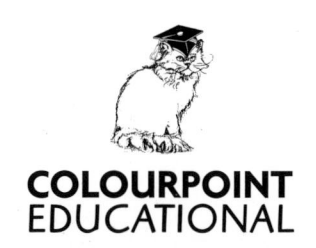

Nora Henry
James Napier
Emma Dougan

COLOURPOINT EDUCATIONAL

© 2019 Nora Henry, James Napier, Emma Dougan and Colourpoint Creative Ltd

ISBN: 978-1-78073-186-5

First Edition
First Impression 2019

Layout and design: April Sky Design
Printed by: W&G Baird Ltd, Antrim

All rights reserved. No part of this publication may be reproduced, stored in a retrieval system or transmitted in any form or by any means, electronic, mechanical, photocopying, scanning, recording or otherwise, without the prior written permission of the copyright owners and publisher of this book.

Copyright

Copyright has been acknowledged to the best of our ability. If there are any inadvertent errors or omissions, we shall be happy to correct them in any future editions.

Front cover: iStockphoto

Images that are copyright to other sources are acknowledged adjacent to the relevant image. All other images are copyright ©Colourpoint Creative Limited.

Colourpoint Educational
An imprint of Colourpoint Creative Ltd
Colourpoint House
Jubilee Business Park
Jubilee Road
Newtownards
County Down
Northern Ireland
BT23 4YH

Tel: 028 9182 6339
E-mail: sales@colourpoint.co.uk
Website: www.colourpoint.co.uk

The Authors

NORA HENRY is a teacher at a Belfast grammar school and a part-time tutor for a university education department. She works for an examining body as Principal Examiner for GCSE Chemistry, Reviser for A level Chemistry and Reviser for A Level Life and Health Sciences. In addition to this text, she has written around 30 textbooks, workbooks and study guides for GCSE and A Level.

JAMES NAPIER is a former teacher at a Northern Ireland grammar school. He has written and co-written a number of Biology and Science textbooks supporting the work of students and teachers. He works for an examining body as Chief Examiner for A Level Biology. He has also published a range of Popular Science books in the areas of Genetics and Evolution. His 'non-science' charity books have raised significant amounts of money for cancer and mental health charities.

EMMA DOUGAN is a Biology lecturer at Southern Regional College and a tutor for a Life Sciences pathway Foundation Degree in Applied Industrial Sciences. She works for an examining body as Principal Examiner for A Level Life and Health Sciences and GCSE Double Award Biology.

Publisher's Note: This book has been through a rigorous quality assurance process by an independent person experienced in the CCEA specification prior to publication. It has been written to help students preparing for the AS Life and Health Sciences specification from CCEA. While Colourpoint Educational, the authors and the quality assurance person have taken every care in its production, we are not able to guarantee that the book is completely error-free. Additionally, while the book has been written to address the CCEA specification, it is the responsibility of each candidate to satisfy themselves that they have fully met the requirements of the CCEA specification prior to sitting an exam set by that body. For this reason, and because specifications and CCEA advice change with time, we strongly advise every candidate to avail of a qualified teacher and to check the contents of the most recent specification for themselves prior to the exam. Colourpoint Creative Ltd therefore cannot be held responsible for any errors or omissions in this book or any consequences thereof.

CONTENTS

Unit AS 2: Human Body Systems

2.1	Cardiovascular system	5
2.2	Respiratory system	15
2.3	Respiration	23
2.4	Homeostatic mechanisms and how these are monitored	29
2.5	Nutrition and physical exercise in maintaining good health	39

Unit AS 3: Aspects of Physical Chemistry in Industrial Processes

3.1	Chemical calculations	53
3.2	Volumetric analysis	59
3.3	Energetics	68
3.4	Kinetics	79
3.5	Equilibrium	85
3.6	Industrial processes	91

Unit AS 5: Material Science

5.1	Material properties	97
5.2–5.3	Categorising materials and microscopic structure	109
5.4–5.5	Alloys, metal working and biomaterials	114
5.6, 5.7, 5.9	Smart materials, nanomaterials and industrial considerations	117
5.8	Semiconductors	123

Answers 126

Unit AS 2:
Human Body Systems

2.1 CARDIOVASCULAR SYSTEM

Students should be able to:

2.1.1 describe the components and functions of the cardiovascular system;

2.1.2 demonstrate an understanding of the histological structure and function of arteries, veins and capillaries;

2.1.3 demonstrate an understanding of the structure and functioning of the heart, to include the phases of the cardiac cycle, myogenic stimulation and the wave of excitation, pressure and volume changes in the heart chambers and major arteries;

2.1.4 demonstrate an understanding of heart sounds and the representation of the excitation wave in an electrocardiogram (ECG), including identifying a normal ECG trace and ECG traces for tachycardia, arrhythmia, ventricular fibrillation and bradycardia heartbeats and how these relate to physiological status; and

2.1.5 describe how to measure pulse rate (the typical range of pulse rate is 60–80 beats per minute) and blood pressure (using a sphygmomanometer), and know normal values for blood pressure for both genders for ages 18–40 years and how changes in these may relate to physiological status.

The cardiovascular system

The key components of the cardiovascular system are:
- blood
- the blood vessels (arteries, veins and capillaries)
- the heart

Blood

The main blood components are the blood cells, platelets and the plasma. The components of the blood have two main functions, these being **transport** and **defence against disease**. The diagram below summarises the key features and roles of the main blood components.

The blood vessels

The three main types of blood vessels are the arteries, veins and capillaries.

Arteries carry blood away from the heart. As these are the blood vessels leaving the heart they carry blood under high pressure and their structure reflects this. The main arteries subdivide to form smaller arteries and arterioles, which in turn subdivide to form capillaries. **Capillaries** have permeable one cell

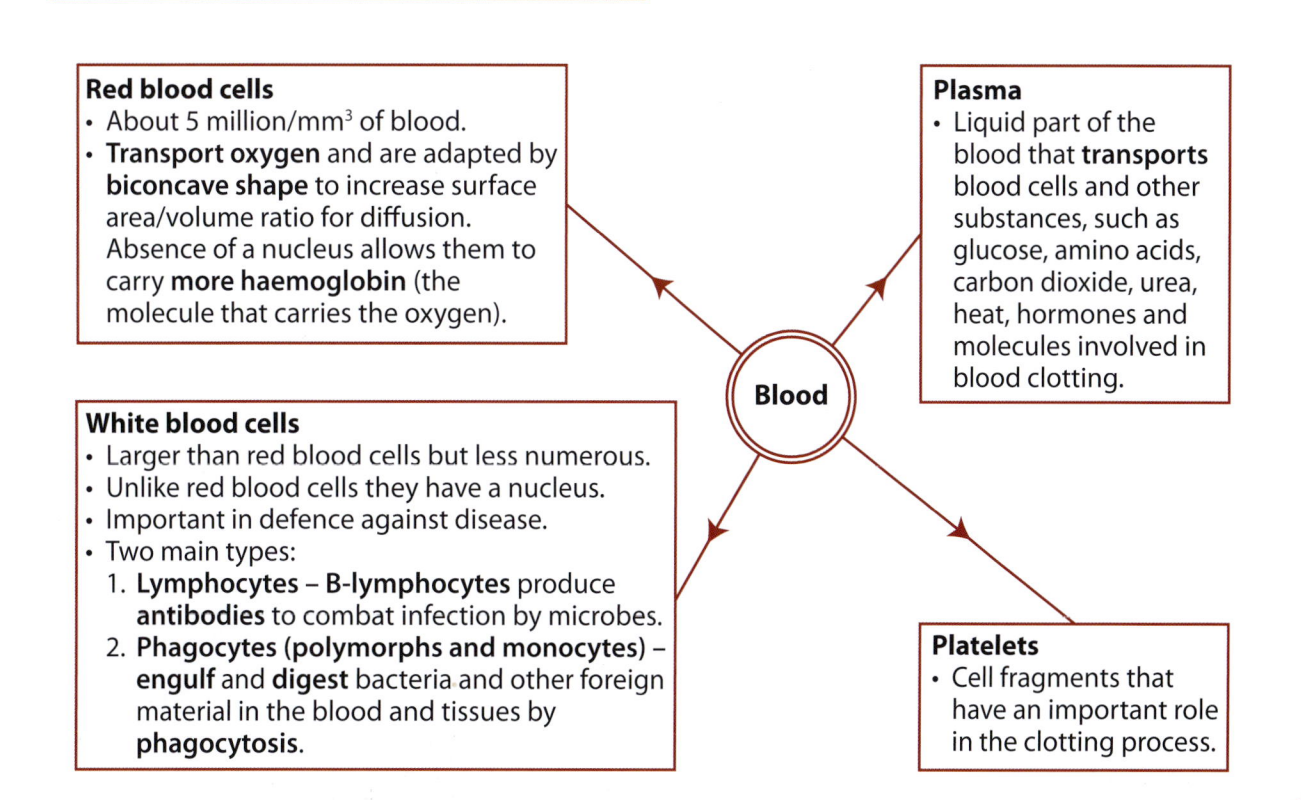

Red blood cells
- About 5 million/mm^3 of blood.
- **Transport oxygen** and are adapted by **biconcave shape** to increase surface area/volume ratio for diffusion. Absence of a nucleus allows them to carry **more haemoglobin** (the molecule that carries the oxygen).

White blood cells
- Larger than red blood cells but less numerous.
- Unlike red blood cells they have a nucleus.
- Important in defence against disease.
- Two main types:
  1. **Lymphocytes** – B-lymphocytes produce **antibodies** to combat infection by microbes.
  2. **Phagocytes (polymorphs and monocytes)** – **engulf** and **digest** bacteria and other foreign material in the blood and tissues by **phagocytosis**.

Plasma
- Liquid part of the blood that **transports** blood cells and other substances, such as glucose, amino acids, carbon dioxide, urea, heat, hormones and molecules involved in blood clotting.

Platelets
- Cell fragments that have an important role in the clotting process.

Blood

thick walls allowing exchange of materials between the blood and tissues. The capillaries eventually merge to form venules, which in turn merge to form small **veins**, which themselves merge to form larger veins that empty their blood into the venae cavae. The structure and function of the main types of blood vessel are summarised in the table below.

Feature	Artery	Vein	Capillary
Structure	• **Thick wall** (an outer thin layer of fibrous tissue, with a thick middle layer of **smooth muscle** and **elastic tissue**, with a thin inner endothelial layer of very thin squamous epithelial cells). • A **narrow lumen**. • Usually an overall **rounded shape**.	• **Thin wall** (an outer thin layer of fibrous tissue, with a thin middle layer containing some muscle and very little elastic tissue, with an inner endothelial layer of squamous cells). • A **large lumen** • **Valves** at intervals along its length. • Much **less regular in shape than an artery**.	• Microscopic vessel with a **one cell thick wall** (consisting of squamous endothelium).
Blood pressure	High (in pulses)	Low	Low
Adaptations	• The **elastic tissue** in the thick middle layer allows the artery to **stretch** as the blood **pulses** out of the heart and through the arteries. • As the **elastic tissue recoils** between heartbeats it helps push blood along the arteries and smooths blood flow. • The **muscle tissue** in the middle layer is essentially a **supporting** layer – it provides strength.	• The **large lumen** offers **little resistance** to blood flow (essential due to low blood pressure in veins). • **Valves** prevent the backflow of blood. There is much **less muscle tissue and elastic tissue** in the walls (again due to the low pressure and the absence of a pulse in veins). • However, as in an artery, a vein has a thin outer protective fibrous layer and an internal endothelial layer of squamous cells.	• Its small size allows an **extensive network** of capillaries, providing a **large surface area** for the diffusion of material. • A capillary has a **very thin wall** (one cell thick) which allows exchange between the blood and the tissues. • The capillary wall is **permeable** to respiratory gases, nutrients such as glucose, and waste including urea, but it is not permeable to large proteins and red blood cells.

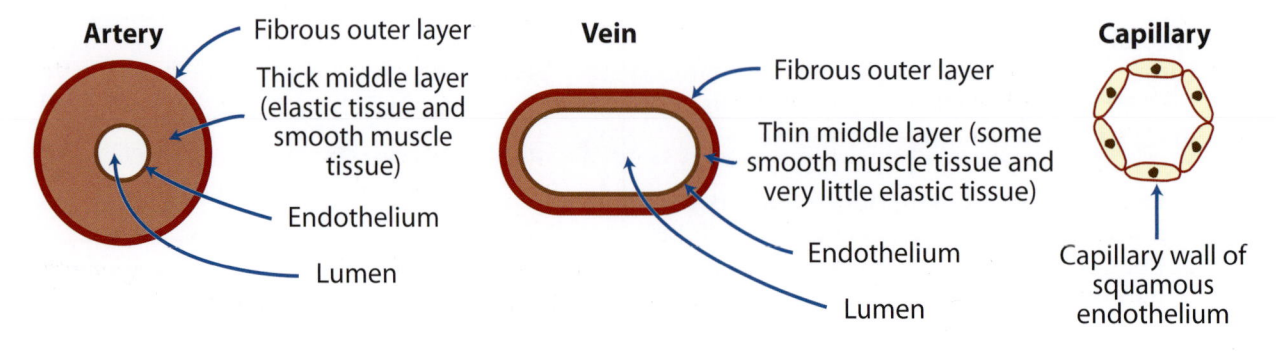

Artery
- Fibrous outer layer
- Thick middle layer (elastic tissue and smooth muscle tissue)
- Endothelium
- Lumen

Vein
- Fibrous outer layer
- Thin middle layer (some smooth muscle tissue and very little elastic tissue)
- Endothelium
- Lumen

Capillary
- Capillary wall of squamous endothelium

Artery, vein and capillary (not to scale)

> **Tip:** The structure of the blood vessels is closely related to the pressure at which they will carry blood. Arteries are adapted for carrying blood at high pressure and veins are adapted for carrying blood at low pressure.

> **Tip:** Note that each of the three types of blood vessel has a thin layer of squamous endothelial cells lining the lumen.

The heart

The heart is the organ that pumps blood through the body. Humans (and other mammals) have a **double circulation**, meaning that the blood travels through the heart twice in each complete circuit of the body. Effectively, this means that there are two distinct circulatory systems – the pulmonary (lung) and systemic (body) systems – with each beat of the heart pumping blood into each system. The right side of the heart pumps blood to the lungs and the left side pumps blood around the body.

The two sides of the heart are separated by a thick muscular wall (the septum) which runs through the centre of the heart.

Heart chambers

Each side has an upper chamber (atrium) and a lower chamber (ventricle). The muscular walls of these chambers are adapted to reflect their respective roles.

- **Atria** – these upper chambers have relatively thin walls, as they receive blood from the lungs (**left atrium**) or the body (**right atrium**) and pump blood into the ventricles that lie directly below them.
- **Ventricles** – these lower chambers have much thicker walls, as they pump blood to the lungs (**right ventricle**) or around the body (**left ventricle**). As the lungs are only a short distance from the heart, the right ventricle does not have to pump blood with the force that the left ventricle does in order to pump blood around the body. Consequently, the right ventricle has less muscular (thinner) walls than the left ventricle.

> **Tip:** You should be able to explain why the walls of the ventricles are thicker than the atria, and why the left ventricle has thicker walls than the right ventricle.

Heart valves

The blood leaves the heart in 'pulses' that coincide with each heartbeat and the heart functions as a one-way pump. Heart valves prevent the blood from flowing back into the atria, as the ventricles contract, and from flowing back into the ventricles from the arteries. There are two types of valves:

- **The atrioventricular (AV) valves** – lie between the atria and the ventricles and prevent the backflow of blood into the atria when the ventricles contract. The valve between the right atrium and right ventricle is sometimes referred to as the **tricuspid** valve and the valve between the left atrium and left ventricle as the **bicuspid** valve.
- **The semilunar (arterial) valves** – lie at the base of the aorta and pulmonary artery and prevent the backflow of blood from the arteries into the ventricles.

The **atrioventricular valves** are anchored by the **papillary muscles** that are embedded in the ventricle wall. **Chordae tendinae** (valve tendons) link the muscles and the valves. These tendons anchor the valves and prevent the valves turning 'inside out' as pressure in the ventricles builds up during contraction.

The **semilunar (arterial)** valves at the base of the arteries close only when the pressure in the arteries exceeds that in the ventricles. When blood is being pumped out of the ventricles they are pushed flat against the artery walls and do not impede flow.

Blood vessels entering and leaving the heart

There are four major blood vessels that enter or leave the heart:

- **The aorta** – is the major **artery** that carries **oxygenated** blood from the **left ventricle**. Arterial branches leading from the aorta carry blood to all the major organs of the body except the lungs.
- **The pulmonary artery** – carries **deoxygenated** blood from the **right ventricle** to the lungs.
- **The venae cavae** – bring **deoxygenated** blood back from the body, returning blood to the **right atrium**.
- **The pulmonary vein** – transports **oxygenated** blood from the lungs to the **left atrium**.

Tip: The pulmonary artery and the pulmonary vein are unusual because the artery carries deoxygenated blood and the vein carries oxygenated blood. They are typical in that they carry blood away from and to the heart respectively, and are histologically (structurally) similar to other arteries and veins.

The diagram below shows the main features of the heart.

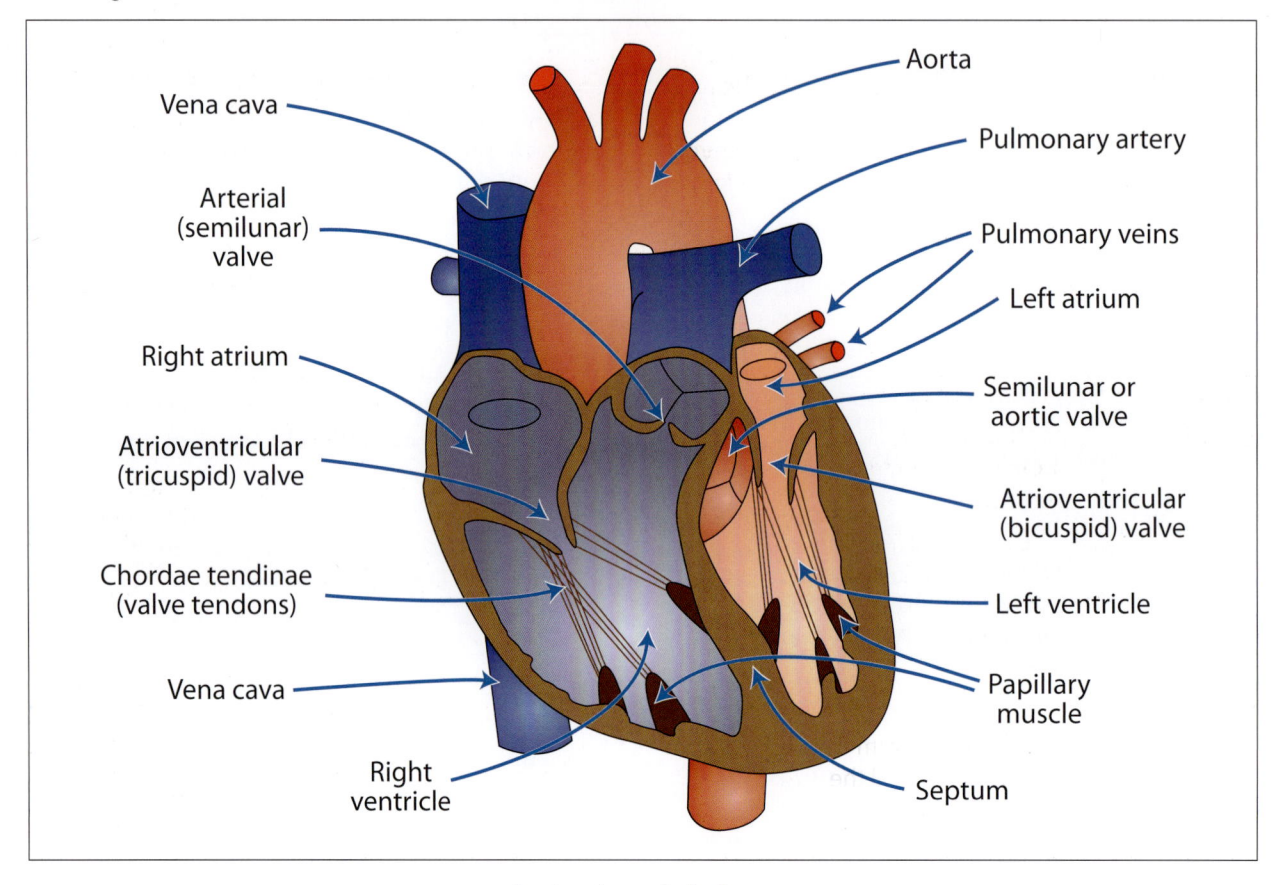

Section through the heart

The **coronary arteries** are arteries that branch off the aorta to supply blood to the heart muscle itself. These can normally be seen running along the outside of the heart surface.

The cardiac cycle

The **cardiac cycle** describes the sequence of events that occur during one heartbeat. This sequence normally occurs between 60–80 times per minute in a human heart. **Diastole** describes a phase when the heart muscle is relaxed and **systole** indicates contraction is taking place. The cardiac cycle has three main stages as described in the table opposite.

2.1 CARDIOVASCULAR SYSTEM

Stage	Atria	Ventricle	Diagram
Diastole	• Atrial walls relax. • Blood enters the atria from the vena cava and the pulmonary vein.	• Ventricle walls also relax. • Semilunar valves close as arterial pressure exceeds the ventricular pressure (due to there being little blood in the ventricles and the ventricles having a larger volume, as the walls are not contracting). • As the AV valves are open, blood enters the ventricles from the atria.	Semilunar valves closed; Vena cava; Pulmonary vein; Blood enters atria and ventricles from vena cava and pulmonary vein; Ventricles relaxed (large volume)
Atrial systole	• Walls of the atria contract forcing more blood into the ventricles. • AV valves remain open as the pressure in the atria still exceeds the pressure in the ventricles. • Blood continues to enter the atria from the vena cava and the pulmonary vein.	• Ventricle walls remain relaxed. • Ventricle volume continues to increase as they fill with blood. • Semilunar valves remain closed.	Semilunar valves remain closed; Atria contract forcing blood into the ventricles; Atrioventricular valves remain open; Ventricles remain relaxed (maximum volume)
Ventricular systole	• Walls of atria relax.	• Ventricle walls contract. • AV valves close as the pressure in the ventricles now exceed the pressure in the atria. • The chordae tendinae prevent the AV valves blowing 'inside out'. • As ventricle pressure reaches its peak, the semilunar valves are forced open, forcing blood into the arteries. • By the end of ventricular systole, the ventricles will be at their smallest volume.	Semilunar valves open; Pulmonary artery; Aorta; Blood pumped out of heart (into pulmonary artery and aorta); Atrioventricular valves close; Ventricles contract (reduced volume)

Pressure changes in the cardiac cycle
The diagram below shows the pressure changes during the cardiac cycle. Stages A–F are summarised below.

A Atrial walls contract (atrial systole), increasing atrial pressure, AV values are open (as atrial pressure > ventricular pressure) and semilunar valves remain closed (as aortic pressure > ventricular pressure).

B Atrial contraction is complete (atria are empty of blood) and ventricles begin to contract (start of ventricular systole). Ventricular pressure > atrial pressure, which leads to AV valves closing **(first heart sounds)**.

C Continued contraction of the ventricles to the extent that ventricle pressure > arterial pressure, resulting in the semilunar valves opening.

D Arterial pressure increases so that arterial pressure > ventricular pressure. This leads to semilunar (arterial) valves closing due to the back pressure **(second heart sounds)**.

E Ventricular pressure falls (little blood present and walls begin to relax). Now, atrial pressure > ventricle pressure, resulting in the AV valves opening.

F Atrial pressure > ventricular pressure as blood is flowing into the atria. AV valves remain open and blood passively flows into the ventricles from the atria.

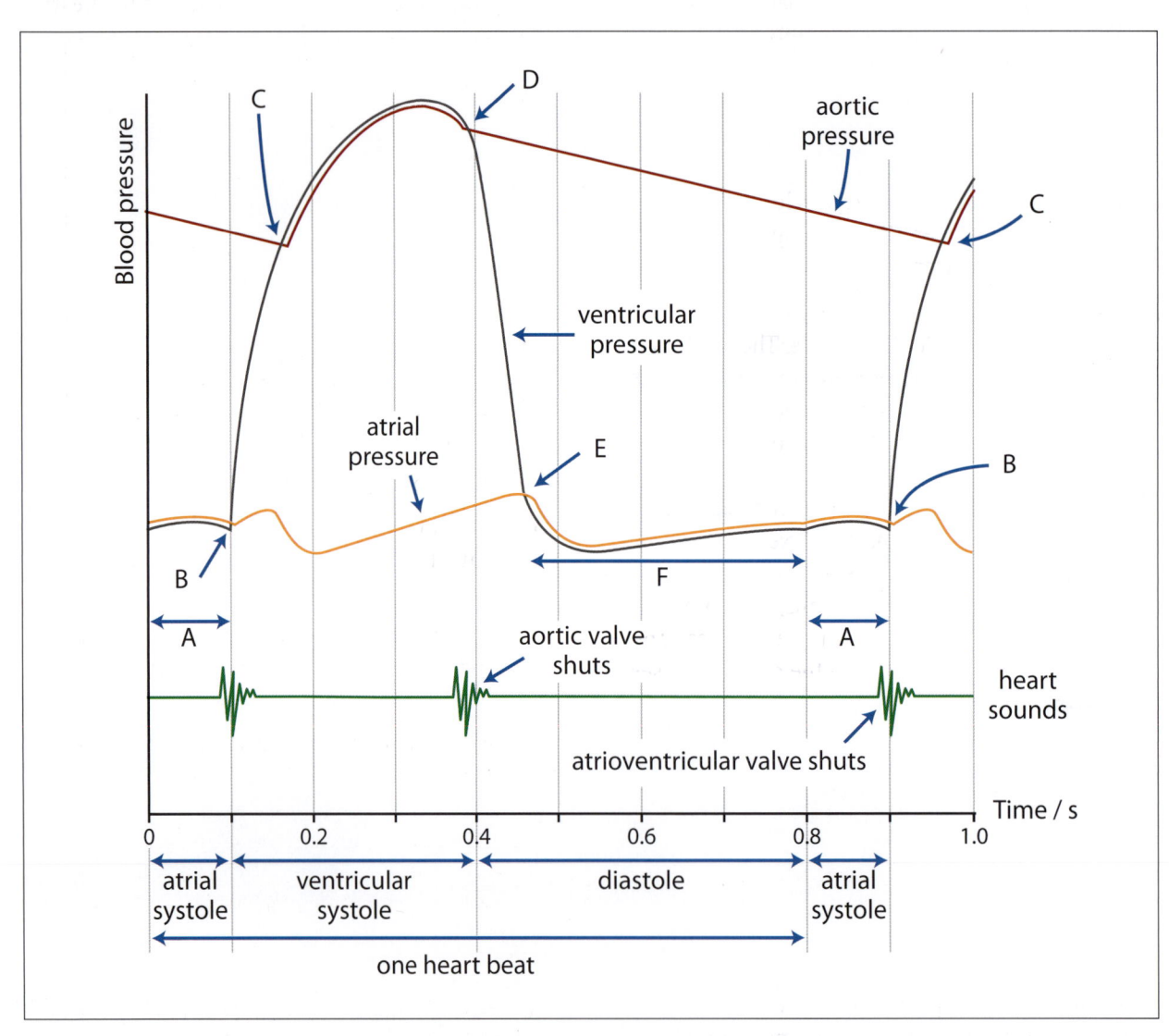

Pressure changes in the left side of the heart during the cardiac cycle (left atrium, left ventricle and aorta). The aortic valve is the semilunar valve at the base of the aorta.

The diagram shows that the atrial pressure rises, falls, then rises again between B and E. This can be explained by:

- the increased pressure of the contracting ventricles causing back pressure against the atria (B–C).
- the subsequent fall in pressure is caused by the relaxation (and increase in volume) of the atria.
- the increase in pressure between 0.2 seconds and E is caused by the atria filling with blood.

Tip: It is important to understand that the heart valves open and close in response to pressure changes either side of the valves (i.e. the AV valves open only if the pressure in the atria exceeds the pressure in the ventricles and close only if the ventricular pressure exceeds the atrial pressure). Valve action is a **response to pressure**; they **do not cause** the pressure changes.

Worked example
State the stages of the cardiac cycle during which the semilunar (arterial) valves open and close. Explain your answer.

Answer
Open during **ventricular systole**. The semilunar valves open when the pressure in the ventricles exceeds the pressure in the arteries (as occurs during ventricular systole) due to the ventricle walls contracting.

Close during **diastole**. Following ventricular systole, the ventricle muscle relaxes and springs out, increasing the volume of the ventricle. As the pressure in the ventricles falls, their pressure drops below the pressure in the arteries. The back pressure from blood in the arteries causes the semilunar valves to close. They remain closed during **atrial systole**.

Coordination of the cardiac cycle and cardiovascular health

Interpreting ECGs
The sequences within the cardiac cycle are stimulated by a coordinated wave of **electrical excitation** through the heart. A small section in the wall of the right atrium acts as a **pacemaker (SA node – sinoatrial node)**, producing electrical signals that pass across the atria walls and then down into and across the ventricles. The **atrioventricular (AV) node** is an area of special tissue in the central wall of the heart (septum) at the junction of the atria and ventricles. It is this node that passes the electrical signal between the atria and the ventricles. Contraction of a particular part of the heart is a consequence of the wave of electrical excitation reaching that part.

Tip: The table of the cardiac cycle (page 9) shows that atrial systole immediately precedes ventricular systole. While this is important in the functioning of the heart, it is controlled by the wave of electrical stimulation passing through the atrial walls before the ventricle walls.

An **electrocardiogram (ECG)** is a graphical representation of the electrical activity in the heart.

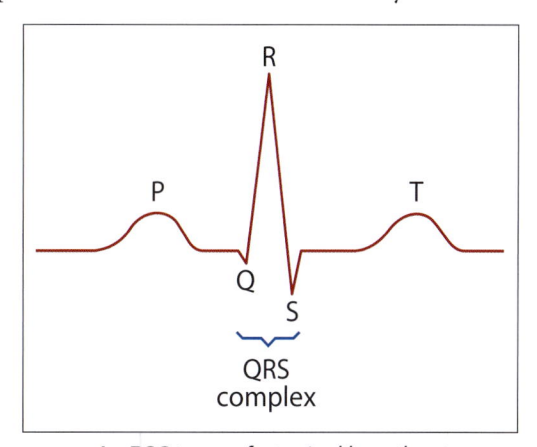

An ECG trace of a typical heartbeat

Key elements of the ECG are:

- the P wave represents the wave of electrical stimulation that triggers the contraction of the atria.
- the QRS complex represents the electrical activity that stimulates contraction of the ventricles.
- the T wave represents the relaxation of the ventricles.

Tip: The R peak has a much greater amplitude than P, as there is much greater electrical activity in the ventricles (reflecting their larger size and thicker muscle).

Tip: The short straight section between the P wave and the QRS complex represents the wave of excitation passing from the atria down into the ventricles.

The table below shows a range of heart traces, displaying normal and irregular heartbeats. The term **arrhythmia** is a general term for a heartbeat problem, meaning the heart is beating irregularly, too fast or too slow.

Heart condition	Trace	Effect
Normal heartbeat		
Bradycardia (heart beating too slowly – typically <60 bpm at rest)		Less blood reaches tissues, therefore there is less oxygen and glucose for respiration. Can cause fatigue, dizziness and fainting.
Tachycardia (heart beating too fast, typically >100 bpm at rest)		Results in rapid pulse rate, palpitations, chest pain, dizziness and fainting. Although the heart is pumping faster it is less efficient and pumps less blood per minute.
Ventricular fibrillation (abnormal rhythm and can indicate a heart attack is taking place)		Very irregular electrical stimulation and the heart contracts in a very uncontrolled and inefficient manner.

Heart sounds

Heart health can also be gauged by the sounds produced by a beating heart. During the cardiac cycle there are two main peaks of sound as identified in the diagram below. These sounds are produced by the atrioventricular and arterial valves closing, as explained earlier.

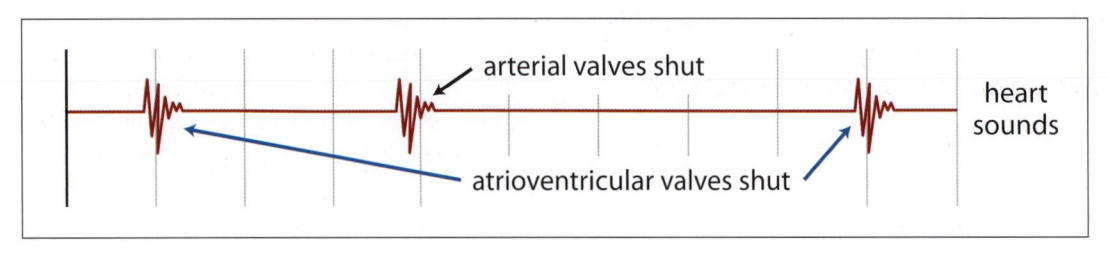

Heart sounds

2.1 CARDIOVASCULAR SYSTEM

Measuring pulse rate and blood pressure

Pulse rate
Pulse rate can be measured manually by feeling for a pulse at a position in the body where an artery is close to the skin, for example, the wrist or neck. The pulse rate can also be measured digitally. For most people, the pulse rate is normally between 60–80 per minute when resting.

Each time the heart beats, a pulse is produced, so pulse rate is effectively heart rate. Pulse rate can change for many reasons, but the most obvious change is when an individual starts exercising. Exercise causes a large increase in pulse rate, as the heart needs to beat more often so that the blood reaches the muscles more quickly (i.e. more blood per unit time) and can deliver the additional glucose and oxygen required for the higher rate of respiration needed.

Blood pressure
Blood pressure is the force produced by the beating of the heart. It can be measured using a **sphygmomanometer**. To measure blood pressure, a cuff is usually placed around the upper arm and inflated to a pressure high enough to stop the blood flow in the artery down the arm.

The pressure in the cuff is reduced slowly until the blood flow (surge) is detected again. This is the **systolic blood pressure** and is usually the upper figure shown in a digital read out. The pressure is reduced further until a constant blood flow is detected. This is the **diastolic blood pressure** and is normally the value on a digital meter just below the systolic value.

While the standard unit (SI) for pressure is the kilopascal (kPa), human blood pressure is traditionally measured in millimetres of mercury (mm Hg). When interpreting blood pressure readings, the upper of the two values is the systolic pressure, which is the blood pressure against the artery walls following ventricular contraction. The lower value is the diastolic pressure, which is the pressure between beats.

Typical values are as shown in the table below.

Age and sex	Typical reading (mm Hg)
18–20 year-old male	125/80
40 year-old male	140/85
18–20 year-old female	120/70
40 year-old female	135/85

In adults, values between **90–130/60–80** are considered normal, with values **>140–90** considered **high** and values **<90–60 low**. However, in general blood pressure **increases with age**.

Blood pressure and lifestyle
Many people have **high blood pressure** (hypertension). Contributing factors include high stress levels, lack of a balanced diet, lack of exercise and hardening of the arteries (arteriosclerosis). Arteriosclerosis reduces elasticity in the artery walls and it can happen as people get older. High blood pressure can be life threatening, as it damages blood vessels and puts a strain on the heart, which can lead to stroke, a heart attack or damage to other organs (such as the kidneys).

A healthy lifestyle is essential to bring blood pressure back to normal long term, although blood pressure tablets are often used. Losing weight, reducing salt intake and exercising are important steps to take to reduce the risk of high blood pressure.

Very **low blood pressure** can also be harmful. It can cause dizziness and fainting, and can be a sign of a failing heart, although it can also be caused by some medicines.

Questions
1. (a) Describe how red blood cells are adapted for their function. [2]
   (b) Describe the passage of the blood and any changes in the blood from when it enters the right atrium (from the venae cavae) until it is pumped out of the left ventricle into the aorta. [4] **[6 marks]**

2. (a) Describe how capillaries are adapted for their function. [3]
   (b) Sections of arteries closer to the heart have more elastic tissue than sections further away from the heart. Explain why. [2] **[5 marks]**

3. (a) Humans have a double circulation. Explain what is meant by this term. [1]
   (b) Describe the process of atrial systole. [2]
   (c) (i) What is meant by the term tachycardia? [1]
       (ii) Give one effect of tachycardia on the body. [1] **[5 marks]**

4. (a) The diagram below shows a blood pressure reading for a 40-year-old man at rest.

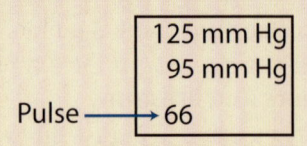

```
            125 mm Hg
             95 mm Hg
   Pulse ──→ 66
```

   (i) What is this man's systolic pressure? [1]
   (ii) Name the condition that this man is suffering from. [1]
   (iii) Name one effect of this condition on the body. [1]
   (iv) Describe how you would use a sphygmomanometer to measure blood pressure. [3]

(b) An individual's pulse rate changed as shown in the table below.

Time/minute	1	2	3	4	5
Pulse rate	68	68	75	98	125

   (i) What is the most likely reason for the change in pulse rate? [1]
   (ii) Explain why the pulse rate changes. [3]

[10 marks]

2.2 RESPIRATORY SYSTEM

Students should be able to:

2.2.1 describe the composition and function of body fluids, to include tissue fluid;

2.2.2. describe the formation of tissue fluid and its return to the circulatory system;

2.2.3 demonstrate an understanding of the chemical composition of haemoglobin in relation to its role in oxygen transport;

2.2.4 demonstrate an understanding of the concept of partial pressure of oxygen and its effect on oxygen transport by haemoglobin;

2.2.5 demonstrate an understanding of the Bohr effect on oxygen transport by haemoglobin and the physiological advantage of this for a tissue;

2.2.6 demonstrate knowledge and understanding of how altitude affects the way haemoglobin transports O_2;

2.2.7 demonstrate an understanding of the structure and functioning of the components of the respiratory system – how these function individually and how the respiratory system functions as a whole – including how they are affected in conditions such as cystic fibrosis and emphysema;

2.2.8 demonstrate an understanding of the factors affecting the rate of gas exchange;

2.2.9 demonstrate an understanding of gas exchange in humans; and

2.2.10 demonstrate an understanding of and explain methods for monitoring the respiratory system – including how to measure breathing rate, tidal volume and vital capacity (using a spirometer) and peak expiratory flow (using a peak flow meter) – knowing average values for these indicators for males and females and how changes in these average values may relate to physiological status.

Body fluids

Living organisms contain a high percentage of water. While all cells contain water, the cells themselves are bathed in what is called **tissue fluid**. Tissue fluid helps keep the cells hydrated but is also important in the nourishment of body cells. Tissue fluid has a well-regulated pH, concentration (to avoid osmotic problems in cells) and ion balance.

Tissue fluid also forms an essential transport link between blood capillaries and the cells. For example, while oxygen is transported in haemoglobin around the cardiovascular system, the red blood cells are too large to exit the capillaries, so the oxygen is released from the haemoglobin in the red blood cells and then diffuses out of the capillary through the tissue fluid and into the cells. Similarly, carbon dioxide produced by respiration in body cells diffuses through the tissue fluid to enter the capillaries before being brought back to the lungs for excretion.

But how is tissue fluid formed? Blood pressure (hydrostatic pressure) forces the liquid part of the blood (all the blood except blood cells and large proteins) through the partially permeable capillary walls and this fluid carries glucose, amino acids, the diffusing oxygen and other substances essential for the cells. This blood plasma essentially becomes the tissue fluid that bathes the cells. This happens much more readily at the arteriole end of the capillary, as at this position the hydrostatic pressure of the blood is relatively high (having just reached the capillaries via the arteries and arterioles). Much of the liquid is then osmotically drawn back into the capillaries and, as this happens, it helps transport the carbon dioxide and other wastes back into them. This is much more likely to occur at the venule end of the capillary, as the plasma in the capillary will be hypertonic compared to the more hypotonic tissue fluid (due to the blood having lost a lot of its liquid at the arteriole end).

The diagram below summarises how tissue fluid is formed.

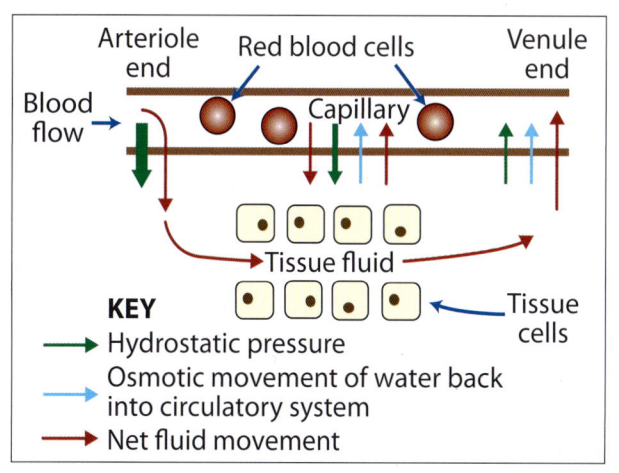

Tissue fluid

There are many other types of body fluids including blood (in which the fluid acts as a transport medium); liquid in the mucus that provides lubrication in the gut; and liquid in the reproductive organs to provide the aqueous medium required for the transport of gametes.

Haemoglobin and oxygen transport

Haemoglobin

Haemoglobin is the protein molecule involved in the transport of oxygen. It is a complex protein consisting of **four polypeptide chains** (two each of two different polypeptides – α and β). Each chain is attached to an **iron-rich haem group**, which is an essential component in terms of oxygen transport.

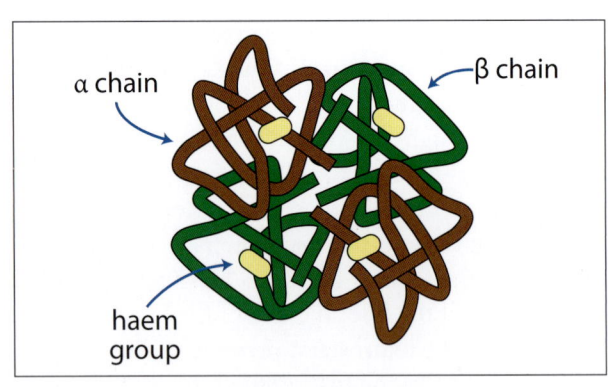

Haemoglobin

Each haem group in the haemoglobin can bind to an oxygen molecule to form **oxyhaemoglobin**. The following equation shows that each molecule of haemoglobin can carry up to four molecules of oxygen.

$$Hb + 4O_2 \rightleftharpoons HbO_8$$
haemoglobin + oxygen $\rightleftharpoons$ oxyhaemoglobin

The equation also shows that the reaction is **reversible**. In conditions where oxygen levels are high, oxyhaemoglobin is formed; if oxygen levels are low the oxygen **dissociates** (breaks free) from the haemoglobin. In mammals, oxyhaemoglobin forms in blood in the lungs where oxygen levels are high (due to gas exchange from the alveoli) and dissociation takes place in the tissues where oxygen levels are low due to respiration using up the available supplies.

> **Tip:** Haemoglobin is highly adapted as a respiratory pigment in that its structure (particularly the presence of the iron-rich haem group) allows it to load and transport oxygen, but also because it is physiologically adapted to load oxygen in high oxygen environments (lungs) and release it in low oxygen environments (tissues).

Haemoglobin normally transports the maximum four oxygen molecules (i.e. it seldom transports one, two or three oxygen molecules only). This increases the efficiency of oxygen transport and is due to the properties of the haemoglobin molecule. When one oxygen molecule is taken up by a haemoglobin molecule, there is a **conformational change** (distortion) in the haemoglobin molecule, resulting in easier (faster) uptake of the remaining three oxygen molecules (**cooperative loading**).

Haemoglobin and oxygen partial pressures

If **every** molecule of haemoglobin in the blood is carrying **four** oxygen molecules, the haemoglobin (blood) is said to be 100% saturated. If only 50% of the haemoglobin is carrying oxygen (assuming they are all carrying four molecules), the blood is 50% saturated and so on.

The degree of saturation of haemoglobin is dependent on the amount of oxygen available in the environment in which the haemoglobin is in at that time. The oxygen concentration in the environment is referred to as its **partial pressure** (pO_2). The partial pressure of any gas is the proportion of total air pressure that is contributed to by that gas and is normally measured in **kilopascals** (kPa).

If haemoglobin molecules are exposed to a range of partial pressures of oxygen, their percentage saturation (with oxygen) can be plotted on a graph known as a **(haemoglobin) oxygen dissociation curve**.

The graph below shows the characteristic **S-shape (sigmoidal)** pattern of oxygen dissociation curves.

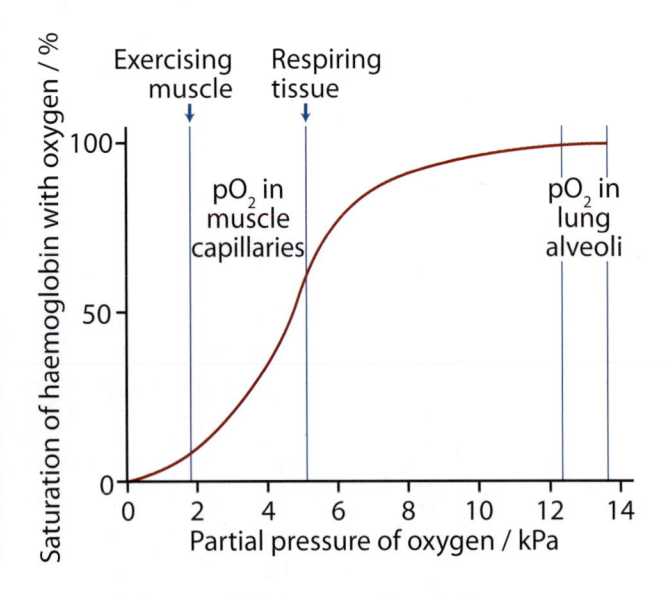

A (haemoglobin) oxygen dissociation curve

Note how in high partial pressures, such as between 12–14 kPa (typically the oxygen partial pressures in the lungs), oxyhaemoglobin is readily formed and the haemoglobin approaches full saturation. The graph shows that the haemoglobin will remain saturated as partial pressures fall only slightly (i.e. the partial pressures associated with the pulmonary vein, the heart, aorta and other arteries).

However, in relatively low partial pressures, such as 2–5 kPa (as found in the tissues), dissociation takes place and the oxygen is released and diffuses into the respiring tissue cells.

The sigmoidal pattern makes the process even more efficient, as over the range of partial pressures typical of respiring tissues there is **rapid dissociation**, making large quantities of oxygen available to the tissues, even though there is a relatively small fall in partial pressure.

The Bohr effect

The physiological ability of haemoglobin to bind with or release oxygen is primarily linked to the partial pressure of oxygen in the environment. However, the **partial pressure of carbon dioxide (pCO_2)** also affects the ability of haemoglobin to combine with oxygen. In higher concentrations of carbon dioxide (i.e. higher than 'normal' levels in the blood), the oxygen dissociation curve moves to the right – **the Bohr effect** (or Bohr shift) – as seen in the graph below.

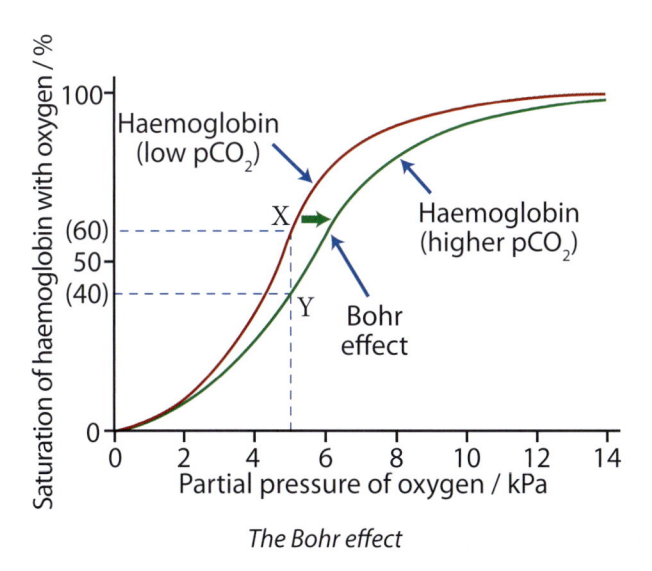

The Bohr effect

The advantage of the Bohr effect is that oxygen is released more readily from haemoglobin at a particular partial pressure of oxygen (i.e. the haemoglobin has a **reduced affinity for oxygen**). In the graph, under normal conditions the haemoglobin is 60% saturated when the pO_2 is 5 kPa (X), meaning that 40% of the oxygen is released to the respiring tissues. With the Bohr effect, at the same partial pressure of oxygen the haemoglobin is only 40% saturated (Y), meaning that 60% of the oxygen transported by the haemoglobin can be released into the tissues.

The Bohr effect occurs when carbon dioxide levels increase, such as when high rates of respiration are taking place (for example, during strenuous exercise). This means that increased oxygen becomes available to the tissues in times of greatest need. Increased blood temperature and a decrease in blood pH also cause the Bohr effect.

> **Tip:** The Bohr effect is not an 'all or nothing' response. The degree of shift to the right depends on the partial pressure of CO_2. The curve will move further to the right if pCO_2 levels are very high, such as during strenuous exercise, as even more rapid oxygen dissociation occurs to match the very high respiration rate that is producing the very high pCO_2.

The effect of altitude on oxygen transport by haemoglobin

As height increases above sea level, overall atmospheric pressure and **pO_2 is reduced**.

The graphs earlier in this section show that if the lungs have a pO_2 environment around 7 kPa, which is typical of very high altitudes (for example, 3500 m above sea level), compared to around 13 kPa in more lowland altitudes, the human haemoglobin cannot become fully saturated and therefore individuals will be able to absorb much less oxygen into their blood.

However, after a period of time living in high altitude, **acclimatisation** can occur. This leads to the body producing an **increase in the number of red blood cells**. To some extent, this compensates for the reduced saturation of haemoglobin in the lower atmospheric pO_2.

> **Tip:** This can explain why many athletes use high altitude training to boost their red blood cell count – an adaptation that would be beneficial whether competing at low or high altitude.

Many populations that have lived at high altitude for **many generations** have evolved a type of haemoglobin that saturates at lower pO_2 levels than typical lower altitude populations.

The human respiratory system and gas exchange

The human respiratory system

The respiratory system ensures that the oxygen required for respiration by body cells reaches the blood (circulatory) system and that excess carbon dioxide is removed.

The diagram below shows the main features of the human respiratory system.

When we breathe in, fresh air rich in oxygen enters through the nose and mouth and passes down the throat into the trachea, bronchi, bronchioles and alveoli. The oxygen diffuses through the alveolar walls into the blood, and carbon dioxide (produced in respiration) diffuses the other way. The pleural membranes lining the lungs and the inside of the chest wall contain pleural fluid that helps to reduce friction as we breathe.

Breathing

Breathing is the term used to describe the processes involved in ventilating the lungs and the alveoli (i.e. bringing oxygen-rich fresh air into the lungs and removing carbon dioxide-rich air).

Inspiration

Inspiration (**inhalation**) describes the process of breathing in. The **external intercostal muscles contract** (as the internal intercostal muscles relax) and the ribs are pulled upwards and outwards. At the same time, the **diaphragm muscle contracts**, causing it to flatten from its domed shape. Both these actions **increase the volume of the thorax** (chest cavity), which in turn **decreases pressure** around the lungs within the thorax. The pressure differential between the atmosphere and the thorax causes **air to enter the lungs** until equilibrium is reached.

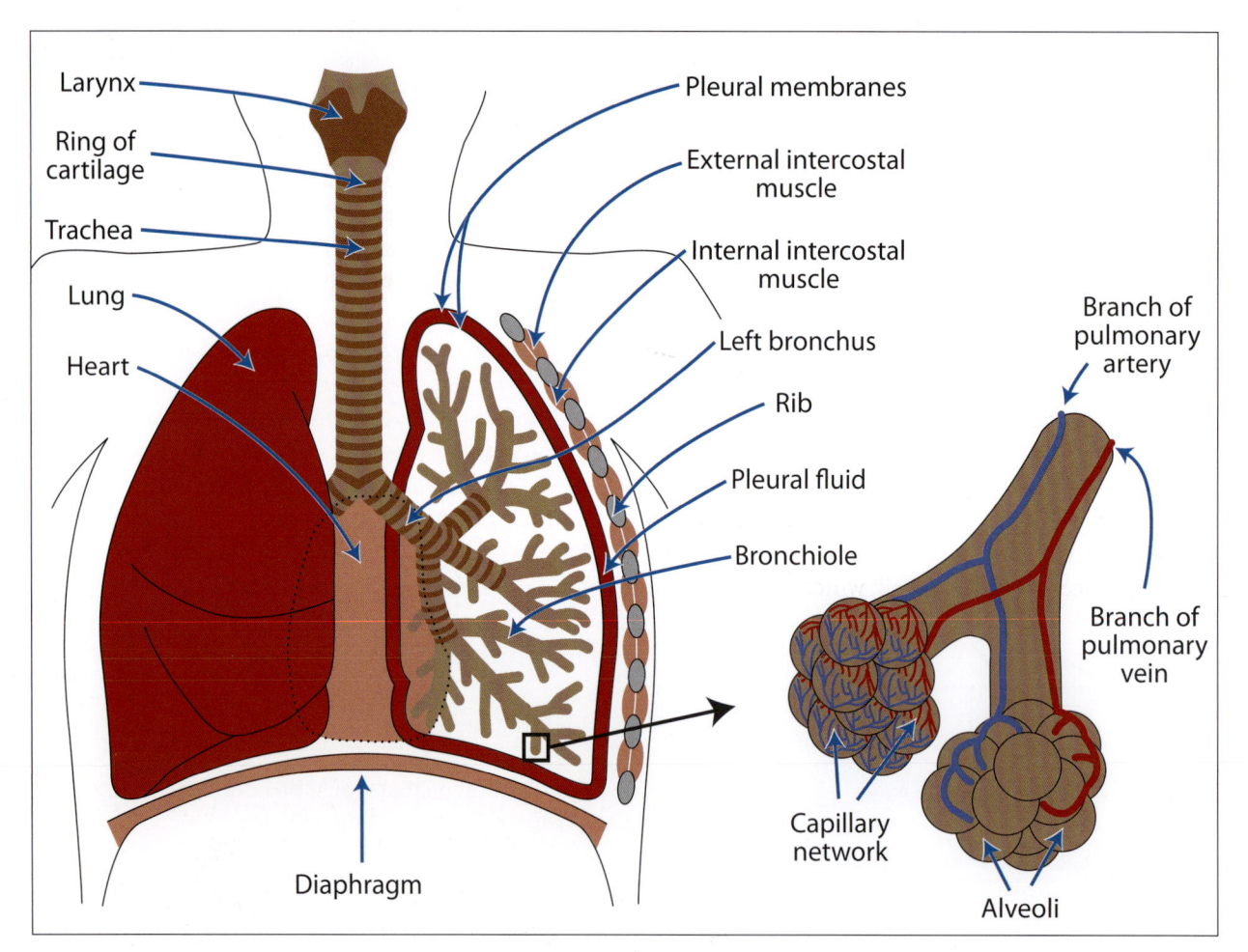

The human respiratory system

2.2 RESPIRATORY SYSTEM

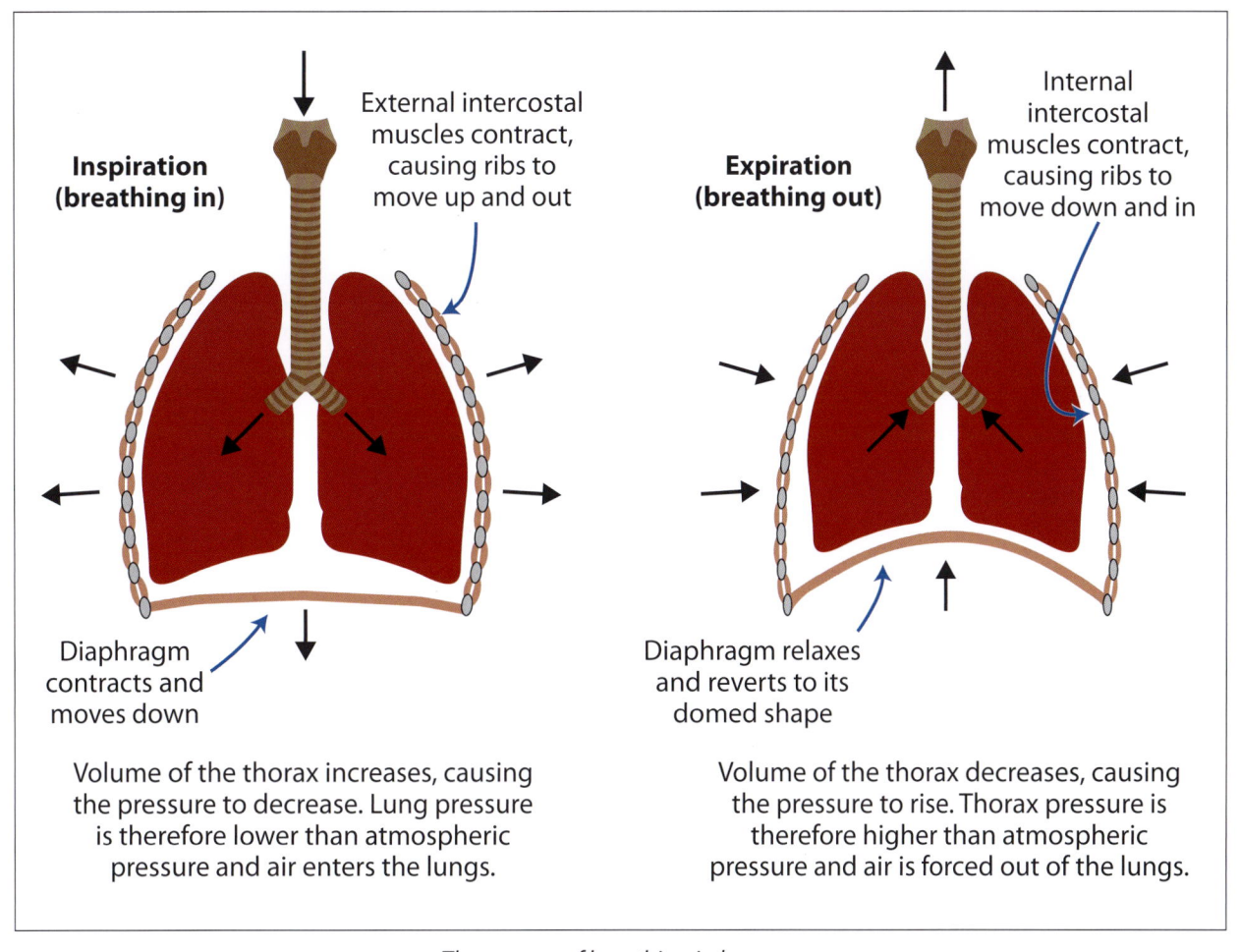

Inspiration (breathing in)
External intercostal muscles contract, causing ribs to move up and out
Diaphragm contracts and moves down
Volume of the thorax increases, causing the pressure to decrease. Lung pressure is therefore lower than atmospheric pressure and air enters the lungs.

Expiration (breathing out)
Internal intercostal muscles contract, causing ribs to move down and in
Diaphragm relaxes and reverts to its domed shape
Volume of the thorax decreases, causing the pressure to rise. Thorax pressure is therefore higher than atmospheric pressure and air is forced out of the lungs.

The process of breathing in humans

Expiration

Expiration (**exhalation**) or breathing out is really the reverse process. The **internal intercostal muscles contract** (as the external intercostal muscles relax), causing the ribs to move down and in. At the same time, the **diaphragm relaxes** and returns to its domed shape. These actions **reduce the volume of the thorax** and **increase the pressure**, forcing **air out of the lungs**. Additionally, the natural elasticity of the lungs produces an elastic recoil, which helps expel air from the lungs.

The diagram above summarises the processes of inspiration and expiration.

Gas exchange

Gas exchange is the term used to describe the movement of respiratory gases in and out of body tissues. In humans (and in other mammals), gas exchange occurs in the walls of the alveoli in the lungs.

Factors that increase the rate of gas exchange:

1. **Large surface area of the exchange surface** – The larger the surface area, the greater the 'surface' across which gases can diffuse. In humans, a large surface area is achieved by having millions of alveoli in the lungs (giving a total gas exchange surface area of around 75 m^2) and also by the rounded shape of each alveolus.

2. **Thin and permeable exchange surface** – Exchange surfaces are thin so that gases can diffuse across. In the alveoli, respiratory gases diffuse in and out of the blood capillaries. Both the alveolar and capillary walls are only one cell thick. These cells are both flattened and in close proximity to each other, so that the overall diffusion distance is very small. The gas exchange surfaces are **moist**, which is essential for gas exchange.

3. **Large concentration gradients** – Diffusion of gases will only occur across an exchange surface

if there is a concentration gradient. Ventilation (breathing) brings oxygen-rich air into the lungs so that the alveoli have a much higher concentration of oxygen than that in the blood. The same principle applies to the removal of carbon dioxide.

> **Worked example**
> Using the diagram below and your knowledge, describe how the lungs are adapted for gas exchange.
>
> Breathing (ventilation) brings oxygen-rich air into alveoli and removes carbon dioxide-rich air
>
> Alveolus
> Capillary
> O_2 CO_2
> Red blood cells in capillary
> Squamous endothelial cells of capillary
>
> **Answer**
> - Alveoli have a large surface area – due to there being many alveoli and the relatively large surface area of each alveolus.
> - There is a very short distance between the alveolus and the capillary.
> - The single layer of flattened cells lining the alveolus and capillary further reduces diffusion distance.
> - Ventilation (breathing) maintains a high concentration gradient between the alveolus and the blood in the capillary (both for oxygen and carbon dioxide).
> - The capillary brings carbon-dioxide rich blood and removes oxygen-rich blood to and from the lungs further increasing the concentration gradient.

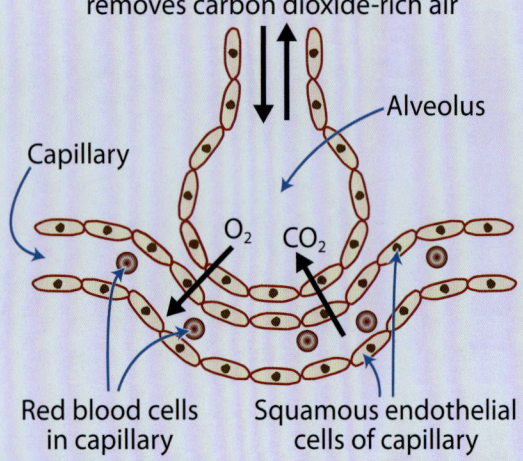

Lung diseases and their effects on gas exchange

Emphysema

Emphysema is a lung condition common in heavy smokers. Irritation from the tar in tobacco smoke damages the alveolar lining to the extent that the walls of many alveoli break down. Fewer alveoli mean that the surface area of the lungs is reduced, resulting in less diffusion of respiratory gases. In addition, tobacco smoke also breaks down the elastic lining of the alveoli, reducing the ability of the alveoli (and lungs) to recoil during expiration, leaving a layer of residual air in the alveoli that prevents fresh inhaled air reaching the gas exchange surfaces. People with emphysema often have increased breathing rates (hyperventilation) in an attempt to compensate for the reduced gas exchange during each breath and they also frequently have an expanded chest.

Cystic fibrosis

Cystic fibrosis is a genetic condition in which affected individuals have two recessive alleles of a particular gene. Affected individuals have more mucus in their respiratory pathway than is normally the case due to the malfunctioning of the CFTR protein, which transports chloride ions in and out of cells. This, and the fact that the build up of mucus makes these individuals more prone to respiratory infections, leads to reduced gas exchange.

Monitoring the respiratory system

The health of the respiratory system can be monitored in many ways, including through the use of peak flow meters and spirometers.

Peak flow meter

Peak expiratory flow (PEF) is an indication of the **force** with which an individual can exhale (breathe out). It is measured using a **peak flow meter** (essentially a small plastic tube with a slider that moves along adjacent to a scale – the greater the force of breathing, the more the slider moves along the scale).

To measure PEF, the subject breathes in deeply and then breathes out as quickly and as hard as possible into the peak flow meter. This causes the slider to move along the scale, with the final

2.2 RESPIRATORY SYSTEM

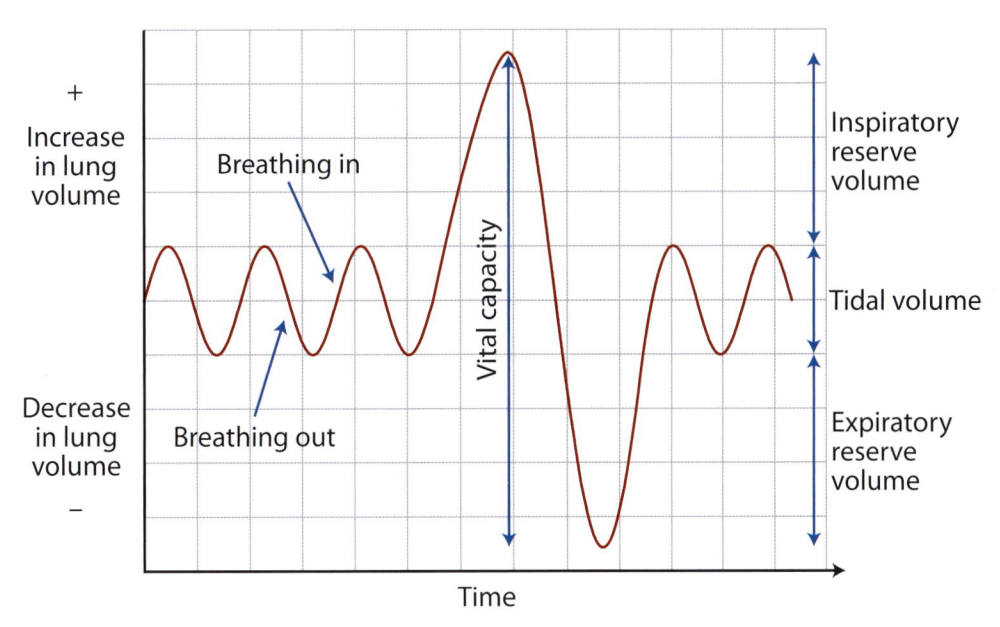

Typical data produced from a spirometer

(maximum) position of the slider representing the PEF value, which can be measured in litres of air breathed out per minute (l/min) or as decimetres^3 per minute (dm^3). One litre = 1 decimetre^3.

PEF peaks in young adults and falls off with age, and men typically have higher values than women. Also, taller/larger people tend to have a higher PEF value than shorter/smaller people. A typical average-sized healthy man of 35 years would be expected to have a PEF value of around **625 l/min**, whereas a typical average-sized woman of 35 years would be expected to have a PEF value of around **430 l/min**.

Breathing in **asthma** sufferers (and individuals with other lung conditions) is typically monitored using a peak flow meter.

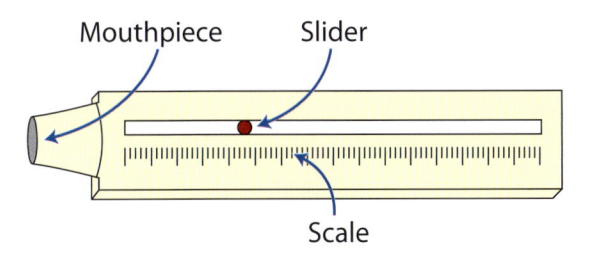

A peak flow meter

Spirometers

A **spirometer** can be used to measure a number of indicators of lung function. It involves breathing into a tube connected to a monitor that provides data such as the individual's **tidal volume** (the amount of air that is normally breathed in and out during ventilation/breathing), their **vital capacity** (the maximum amount of air that can be breathed out following a maximum inhalation) and **breathing rate** (number of breaths per minute), as represented in the graph above. The **inspiratory reserve volume (IRV)** is the maximum amount that can be breathed in above and beyond normal tidal inspiration and the **expiratory reserve volume (ERV)** is the maximum amount that can be breathed out above and beyond the normal tidal expiration.

Spirometers can be used to monitor many lung conditions, including chronic obstructive pulmonary disease (COPD). It provides a greater range of data than a peak flow can give.

Typical values are shown in the table below.

	Male	Women
Breathing rate	12–18	12–18
Tidal volume	500 (ml)	390 (ml)
Vital capacity	3.5–6 (l)	2.5–4.7 (l)

Questions

1. (a) Describe how haemoglobin is adapted to maximise oxygen transport. [2]
   (b) (i) Describe what is meant by the term 'partial pressure of oxygen'. [1]
   (ii) Describe what is meant by the Bohr effect and explain its benefit during periods of extensive muscular activity. [4]   **[7 marks]**

2. (a) Explain the process of inspiration (breathing in) in humans. [3]
   (b) (i) A high concentration gradient helps increase gas exchange. State two ways in which high concentration gradients in the lungs are achieved, thus maximising the exchange of oxygen from the alveoli into the blood. [2]
   (ii) State two other factors that are important in gas exchange. [2]

   [7 marks]

3. (a) The graph below shows typical peak expiratory flow (PEF) values for a 'typical' man and an 'typical' woman of average size.

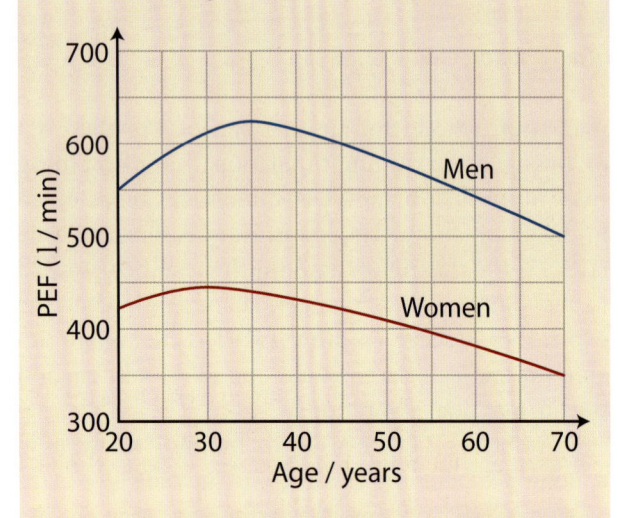

   (i) Compare and contrast the PEF values for men and women. [2]
   (ii) Suggest possible explanations for the change in PEF values in men with age. [2]
   (b) Spirometers can measure tidal volume and vital capacity.
   (i) Explain what is meant by the terms tidal volume and vital capacity. [2]
   (ii) People with emphysema normally have a higher breathing rate than those without the condition. Explain why. [2]

   [8 marks]

2.3 RESPIRATION

Students should be able to:

2.3.1 describe the role that breathing plays in cellular respiration;
2.3.2 demonstrate an understanding that respiration involves chemical reactions that use oxygen;
2.3.3 describe how adenosine triphosphate, ATP, is produced by the process of aerobic respiration;
2.3.4 recognise the nature and function of ATP;
2.3.5 demonstrate an understanding of glycolysis;
2.3.6 demonstrate an understanding of aerobic respiration;
2.3.7 demonstrate an understanding of the Krebs cycle;
2.3.8 demonstrate an understanding of the electron transport chain;
2.3.9 demonstrate knowledge and understanding of anaerobic respiration to include glycolysis and further reactions that produce no more ATP but regenerate NAD and lactate production;
2.3.10 compare aerobic and anaerobic respiration; and
2.3.11 define what is meant by basal metabolic rate (BMR).

Cellular respiration and ATP

Cellular respiration

Cellular respiration is the term that describes the release of energy from food in body cells. The word equation for respiration is:

oxygen + glucose → carbon dioxide + water + energy (ATP)

As can be seen in this equation, oxygen and glucose (carbohydrate) are used to produce energy with water and carbon dioxide as waste products. Respiration in the presence of oxygen is referred to as **aerobic respiration**. While the actual process of respiration takes place in cells, it is the process of breathing that provides the body cells with oxygen and removes the excess carbon dioxide produced.

Tip: Do not confuse breathing with respiration – breathing is a process that brings oxygen into the lungs (oxygen that eventually reaches the body cells) and removes excess carbon dioxide. The actual reactions of respiration take place in body cells (cellular respiration).

Adenosine triphosphate (ATP)

Adenosine triphosphate (ATP) is the molecule produced in cellular respiration. ATP has **three phosphate groups** combined with the nucleotide base **adenine** and a **ribose** sugar, as shown in the diagram below.

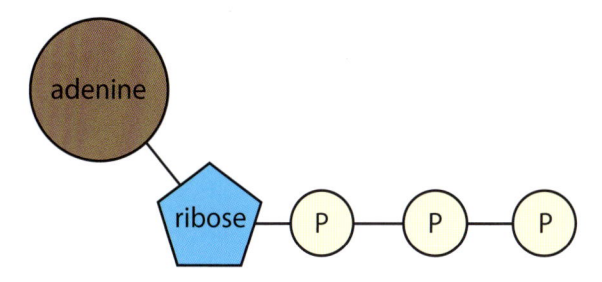

The structure of ATP

ATP is the **immediate source of energy** (the energy 'currency') in a cell. It is the ATP that provides the energy for metabolism and any body process requiring energy (for example, muscle contraction).

Tip: Metabolism is the sum of all the reactions that take place in the body – (cellular) respiration is only one of the very many reactions that take place in a cell.

ATP is synthesised from **ADP** (adenosine diphosphate), a molecule with two phosphate groups and **inorganic phosphate** (P_i) as shown in the diagram below.

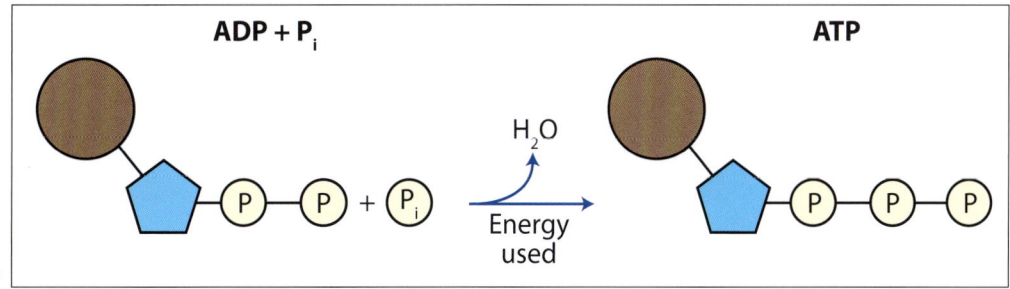

The formation of ATP

The release of energy from ATP

The process of forming ATP from ADP and inorganic phosphate is known as **phosphorylation** (the addition of phosphate to a molecule) and the effect is to make the molecule with the extra phosphate (ATP) more energy rich.

When the third phosphate is removed (as shown in the diagram above), energy is released that can then drive the metabolic reactions in the cell.

> **Tip:** ATP has many advantages in its role as the energy 'currency' – the breakdown of ATP releases small, manageable amounts of energy within cells. Only a single reaction is involved, indicating that energy can be released quickly. It is also a small soluble molecule that can be easily transported around cells.

The biochemistry of aerobic respiration

In mammals, the principal respiratory substrate is glucose. Therefore, respiration is essentially the conversion of glucose into ATP. In humans and other mammals, respiration normally involves the utilisation of oxygen and is therefore referred to as aerobic respiration. There are four main stages of aerobic respiration:

1. **Glycolysis** – the splitting of 6-carbon glucose into two 3-carbon pyruvate molecules.
2. **Link reaction** – the conversion of pyruvate into 2-carbon Acetyl-CoA.
3. **Krebs cycle** – the feeding of Acetyl-CoA into a cyclical series of reactions that produces hydrogen atoms which are used in the electron transport chain.
4. **Electron transport chain** – the process during which most of the ATP in cellular respiration is produced.

Glycolysis

Glycolysis is the first step in cellular respiration. The initial stage is the **activation** of glucose by phosphorylation – this means that ATP is added to glucose to make it more reactive. The addition of the phosphates converts the glucose into **fructose bisphosphate**.

The fructose bisphosphate **splits into two** 3-carbon molecules of **triose phosphate**. The triose phosphate is oxidised through the loss of hydrogen atoms to form **pyruvate**. The hydrogen atoms released to cause the oxidation are collected by the hydrogen carrier molecule **NAD**, which becomes reduced to form **reduced NAD** or **NADH**. The removal of hydrogen involves dehydrogenase enzymes in a process called **dehydrogenation**.

In converting **each** molecule of triose phosphate into a pyruvate molecule, **two ATP molecules** are produced, therefore giving **glycolysis a net gain of two ATP**.

> **Tip:** As each of the triose phosphate molecules produce two ATP (and remembering that one glucose molecule splits to form two triose phosphate molecules), four ATP are produced in total. This gives a net gain of two ATP (as two ATP were initially used to activate the glucose).

> **Tip:** Several stages in respiration involve oxidation and reduction (redox) reactions. The loss of hydrogen atoms from a molecule oxidises the molecule that loses the hydrogen (oxidation) and the molecule (a hydrogen carrier) receiving the hydrogen becomes reduced (reduction). When a molecule becomes reduced it gains energy and when it becomes oxidised it loses (releases) energy.

> **Tip:** The process of glycolysis does not require oxygen.

2.3 RESPIRATION

The diagram below summarises the process of glycolysis.

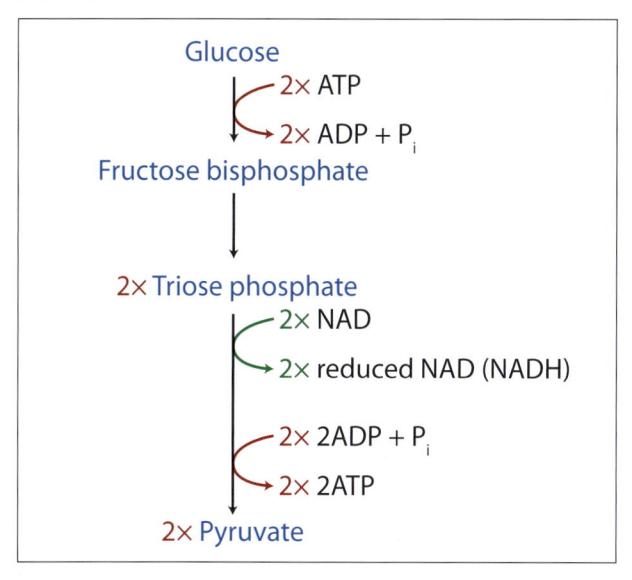

```
Glucose
  │ ⤷ 2× ATP
  │ ⤶ 2× ADP + P_i
Fructose bisphosphate
  │
  ↓
2× Triose phosphate
  │ ⤷ 2× NAD
  │ ⤶ 2× reduced NAD (NADH)
  │ ⤷ 2× 2ADP + P_i
  │ ⤶ 2× 2ATP
2× Pyruvate
```
Glycolysis

Link reaction
During the link reaction, the pyruvate produced in glycolysis is converted to the 2-carbon **Acetyl-CoA**. One molecule of **carbon dioxide** is released during this reaction (this accounts for a 3-carbon molecule – pyruvate – being converted into a 2-carbon molecule) and hydrogen is released during a dehydrogenation reaction to convert **NAD to NADH**.

Krebs cycle
The Krebs cycle is a cyclical series of reactions during which:
- **carbon dioxide is released at two points** (during the conversion of a 6-carbon compound to a 5-carbon compound and then to a 4-carbon compound).
- at **three points** in the cycle, hydrogen is released that converts **NAD to NADH**.
- at **one point**, the hydrogen acceptor (carrier) is not NAD but a related molecule **FAD**, which forms **FADH$_2$**.
- at **one point**, ATP is produced directly (by the transfer of phosphate from an intermediate compound in the cycle to ADP). ATP produced in this way is referred to as **substrate-level (substrate-linked) phosphorylation**.

The Krebs cycle is summarised in the diagram below.

> **Tip:** As there are two molecules of Acetyl-CoA formed for every molecule of glucose, there will be two turns of the cycle for each glucose molecule.

The electron transport chain
Essentially, the electron transport chain uses the hydrogen atoms collected by NAD and FAD to pass through a series of hydrogen carriers that undergo a series of oxidation-reduction reactions to form ATP. Part of the way along the chain, hydrogen atoms split to form electrons and protons – from this point on it is electrons that cause the reduction of the carriers (and why the chain is referred to as electron transport rather than hydrogen transport).

The electron transport chain is a series of hydrogen or electron carriers arranged in a way that hydrogen or electrons can pass from carrier to carrier, reducing the carriers that accept them and oxidising those that release them. Energy becomes available as these

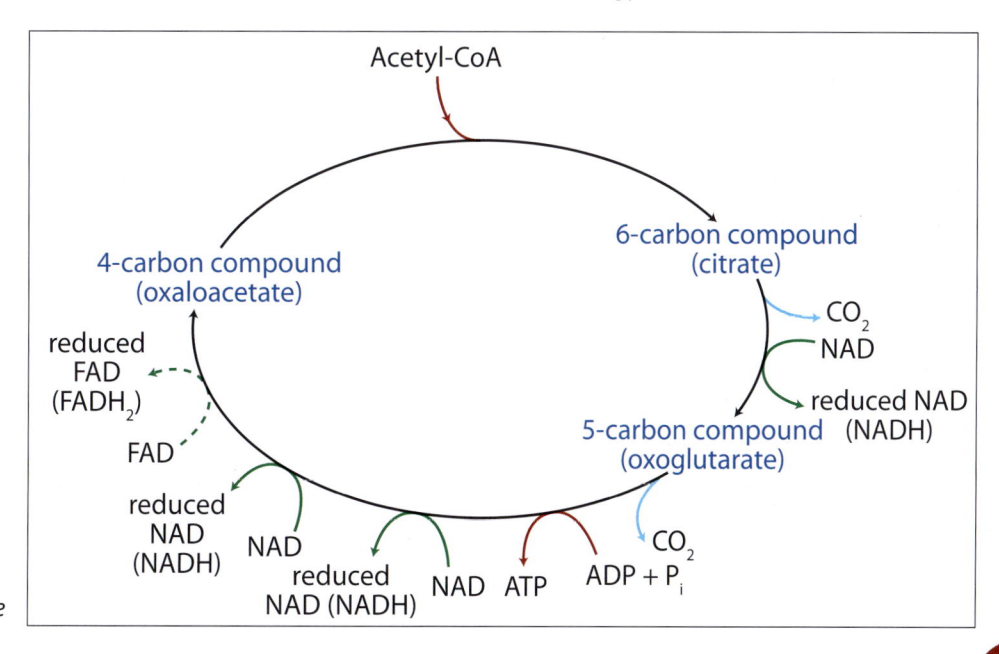

The Krebs cycle

redox reactions take place. At certain points there is enough energy to produce ATP by **oxidative phosphorylation**.

The diagram below shows that when NAD is reduced to **NADH**, **three ATP** molecules are produced, but when FAD is reduced to **FADH$_2$**, only **two ATP** are produced.

The diagram also shows that the electrons recombine with their protons at the end of the chain to form hydrogen, which combines with **oxygen** to form **water** as a waste product. For this reason, oxygen can be referred to as the **final hydrogen (electron) acceptor**.

> **Tip:** The production of ATP in the electron transport chain is referred to as **oxidative phosphorylation**, as oxygen is used as part of the process.

> **Tip:** Remember that NAD becomes reduced (to form NADH) by hydrogen atoms being released by reactions during glycolysis, the link reaction and Krebs cycle (and FAD is also reduced by hydrogen released in Krebs).

> **Tip:** Remember also that two triose phosphate molecules are produced from one molecule of glucose, therefore every stage after the production of triose phosphate can be counted twice in terms of the ATP produced or NAD/FAD reduced per glucose molecule (this includes the link reaction, Krebs cycle and the electron transport chain).

How much ATP is produced in aerobic respiration?

ATP is produced directly (substrate-linked phosphorylation) and by the electron transport chain (oxidative phosphorylation) as a result of hydrogen atoms becoming available from reactions. In total **38 ATP** are produced from the respiration of one molecule of glucose.

Worked example
Explain how 38 ATP molecules are produced from one glucose molecule in aerobic respiration.

Answer
4 ATP are produced by substrate-level phosphorylation (a net gain of 2 in glycolysis and 2 in the Krebs cycle).

30 ATP are produced in the electron transport chain as a result of **10** NAD molecules being reduced (6 in Krebs; 2 in glycolysis; 2 from the link reaction).

4 ATP are produced in the electron transport chain as a result of FAD being reduced.

The electron transport chain

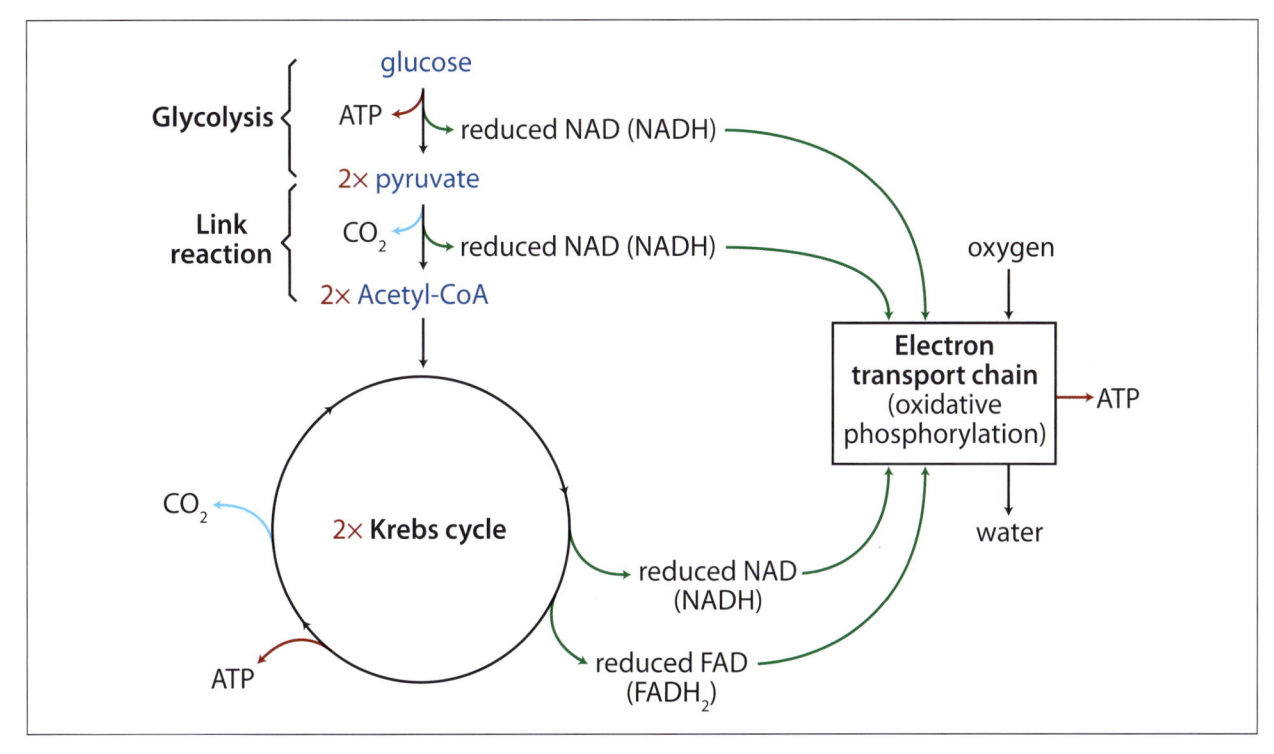

Summary of the biochemistry of aerobic respiration

Where do the various stages of respiration take place?

The initial stage of respiration (glycolysis) takes place in the cell **cytoplasm**.

However, pyruvate (the final product of glycolysis) is transported into a special organelle in the cell called the **mitochondrion**. The remaining stages (and production of 36 of the 38 ATP) take place in the mitochondrion. The link reaction and Krebs cycle take place in the **matrix** (the main body of the mitochondrion) and the electron transport chain takes place in a specialised inner membrane of the mitochondrion that is highly folded to form **cristae**.

Summary of the biochemistry of aerobic respiration

The diagram above summarises the different stages of aerobic respiration.

Anaerobic respiration

When oxygen is not available, **anaerobic respiration** can take place in muscles for short periods of time.

Although oxygen is only used at the end of the electron transport chain, without it the link reaction, Krebs cycle or the electron transport chain do not take place.

Glycolysis is the only ATP-producing stage of anaerobic respiration; therefore, there is a net gain of **two ATP** from the respiration of one molecule of glucose.

In anaerobic respiration, glycolysis will only continue if its products are removed and not allowed to accumulate. The pyruvate is converted to **lactate** (which will eventually be broken down). The reduced NAD (NADH) is oxidised as its hydrogens are used in the reactions that form lactate from pyruvate. This process provides the necessary NAD molecules for 'mopping up' the hydrogen released during glycolysis. Anaerobic respiration is summarised in the diagram below.

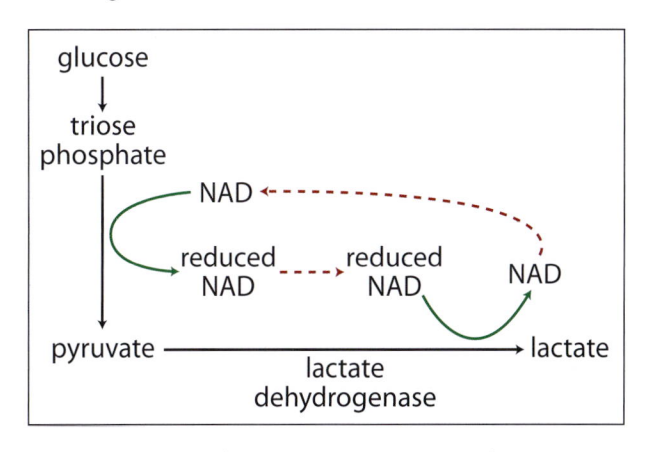

Anaerobic respiration in mammals

Although anaerobic is not very efficient, for short periods of time it can produce **extra ATP** above and beyond what can be produced in aerobic respiration. However, after a period of time respiring anaerobically, the lactate can build up to cause cramp.

> **Tip:** Anaerobic respiration in mammals produces much less ATP than aerobic respiration and it produces only lactate as a waste product (rather than water and carbon dioxide).

Basal metabolic rate

Metabolic rate describes the sum total of activity in our body in terms of processes such as cellular respiration, digestion, breathing and tissue repair.

Our metabolic rate varies considerably. For example, it will obviously be much higher when we are running than when we are sleeping.

However, there is a minimum amount of activity in our body just to 'tick over' when we are completely at rest. This minimum level of activity is referred to as the **basal metabolic rate (BMR)**. We very seldom, if ever, have this baseline level of activity – we would need to be sitting motionless, at a time long enough after a meal to have all the food digested and absorbed, but not hungry (as stress uses more energy), and in a room temperature that does not require us to increase or decrease heat loss.

In mammals, metabolic rate can be compared by measuring heat produced per unit of surface area over time, or indirectly, through oxygen consumption using a spirometer.

Questions

1. (a) Explain the difference between breathing and respiration. [4]
   (b) Describe what is meant by the term basal metabolic rate (BMR). [1] **[5 marks]**

2. (a) Name the components of ATP. [1]
   (b) Describe fully how ATP is formed. [2]
   [3 marks]

3. (a) The diagram below summarises the Krebs cycle.

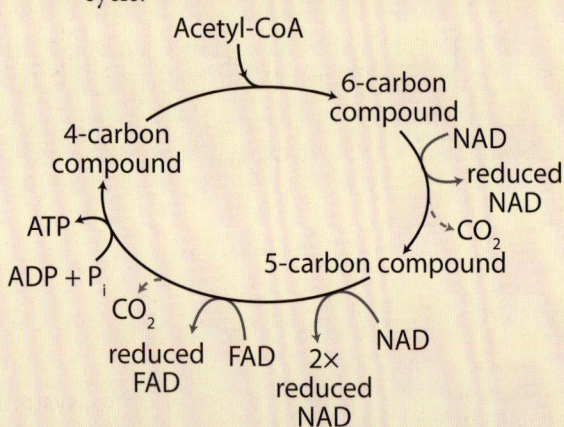

   Acetyl-CoA → 6-carbon compound → (NAD → reduced NAD, CO_2) → 5-carbon compound → (CO_2, reduced FAD, FAD, 2× reduced NAD, NAD) → 4-carbon compound → (ATP, ADP + P_i) → (back to cycle)

   Use the diagram and your knowledge to answer the following questions.
   (i) How many molecules of ATP are produced by substrate-level phosphorylation from one turn of the Krebs cycle? [1]
   (ii) At several points during the Krebs cycle, dehydrogenation takes place and hydrogens are taken up by hydrogen acceptors. Explain the significance of this in ATP production. [3]
   (iii) The diagram shows that two molecules of carbon dioxide are given off during one turn of the Krebs cycle. Explain how the aerobic respiration of one molecule of glucose produces six molecules of carbon dioxide. [3]
   (b) Name the part of the mitochondrion in which the Krebs cycle takes place. [1]
   [8 marks]

4. Anaerobic respiration is much less efficient than aerobic respiration in terms of ATP production.
   (a) How many ATP are produced from one molecule of glucose in anaerobic respiration? [1]
   (b) Give one advantage of anaerobic respiration in humans. [1]
   (c) Apart from ATP, give one other product of anaerobic respiration in humans. [1]
   [3 marks]

2.4 HOMEOSTATIC MECHANISMS AND HOW THESE ARE MONITORED

Students should be able to:

2.4.1 describe the concept of homeostasis and the components of homeostatic mechanism;

2.4.2 describe the role of hormones in body function;

2.4.3 describe the regulation and monitoring of blood glucose levels – including the actions of insulin and glucagon – and the effects of food intake, physical activity and diabetes on insulin, glucagon and blood glucose levels;

2.4.4 explain the source, role and control of thyroxine;

2.4.5 demonstrate an understanding of the homeostatic mechanisms involved in the regulation of sodium;

2.4.6 explain the importance of sodium ions and chloride ions in the healthy functioning of the body;

2.4.7 explain how blood is buffered to maintain normal blood pH range (7.35–7.45) and how blood pH is monitored;

2.4.8 describe the causes and consequences of blood becoming acidic or alkaline; and

2.4.9 demonstrate an understanding of and explain the monitoring of oxygen saturation (SpO$_2$%; normal levels 94–99%) by pulse oximeter, how oxygen saturation is affected by blood pH and temperature, and the conditions that may lead to reduced SpO$_2$% levels, including cystic fibrosis, emphysema and pneumonia.

Homeostasis

Homeostasis is the maintenance of **constant** or **steady state** conditions within the body.

In mammalian tissues, cells are surrounded with tissue fluid. The tissue fluid contains a range of substances from the blood. The composition of tissue fluid and blood must be kept constant or within narrow limits, irrespective of the external conditions outside the body, for cells to function properly.

There are a number of factors that are kept **constant** by homeostasis, such as body temperature, blood glucose levels, blood pH, water and ion content.

Most **homeostatic mechanisms** involve the following components:

- A **stimulus** that causes a change in the factor being controlled.
- A **control system** with **receptors** (sensors) that **detect** the change in the factor being controlled. The receptors may be in the brain or located throughout the body. The control centre is normally the brain; the receptors provide information allowing the control system to **monitor** the factor being controlled.
- An **effector** that causes a **response** and brings about a **corrective mechanism** to return the factor to its **normal** level (set point).

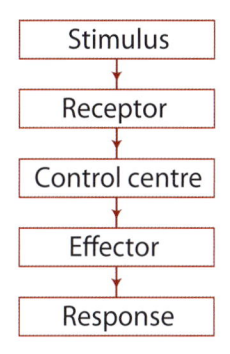

Components of a homeostatic mechanism

The corrective mechanism involves a **negative feedback** system. Negative feedback occurs when the factor being controlled returns to its normal level (set point). As a result, the corrective measures are turned off. This prevents over-correction.

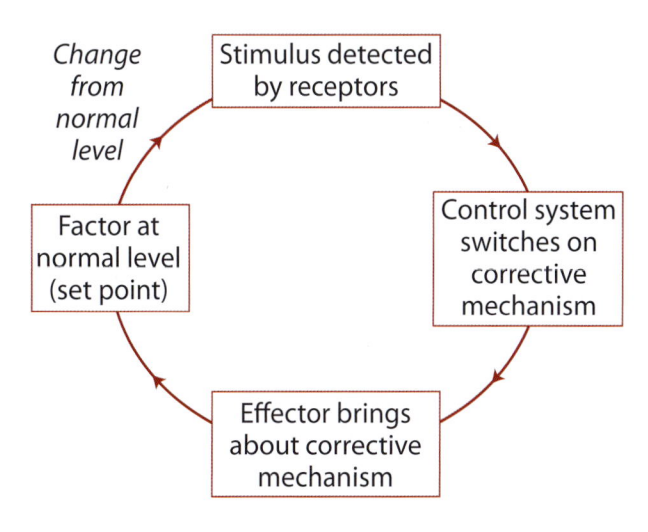

Negative feedback

Tip: You may be given an example of a negative feedback mechanism that you have not already encountered, and be expected to recognise it as such.

The role of hormones in body function

A hormone is a **chemical** substance, produced by an **endocrine gland**. Hormones are released into the **bloodstream** and travel to a **target** organ or target cells. Hormones play an essential part in the body's **communication** system. In comparison to a **nervous** response, hormones produce a **slower, longer-lasting** and more **widespread** response.

Tip: Hormones target particular cells. The target cells have **specific receptor proteins** with a binding site that has a **complementary shape** to the shape of the hormone.

The **endocrine system** is made up of all the endocrine glands in the body. These are shown in the diagram opposite.

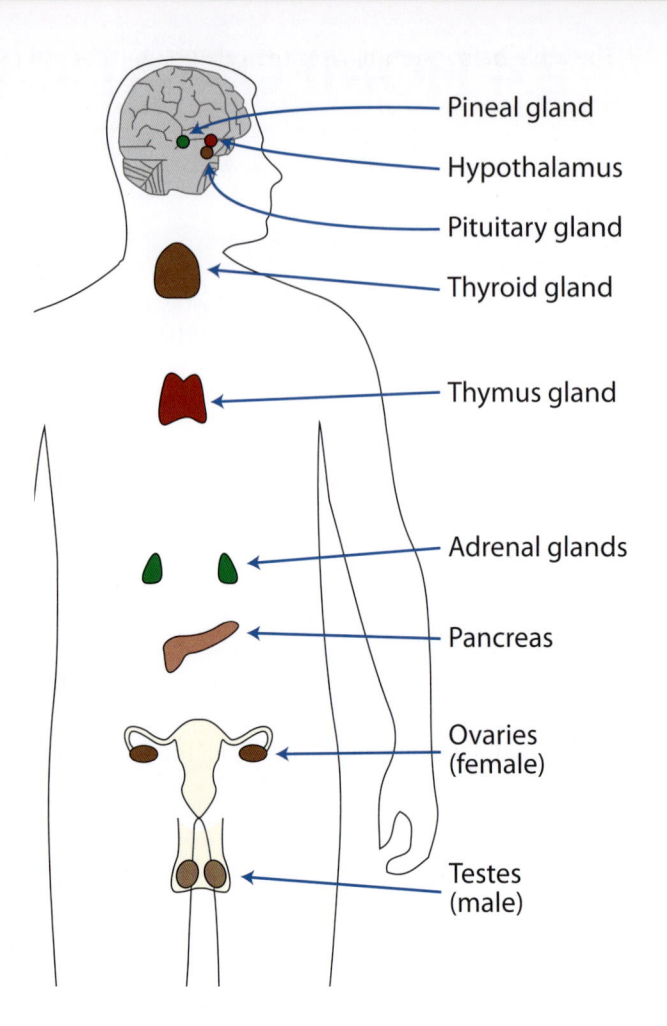

- Pineal gland
- Hypothalamus
- Pituitary gland
- Thyroid gland
- Thymus gland
- Adrenal glands
- Pancreas
- Ovaries (female)
- Testes (male)

Glands of the endocrine system

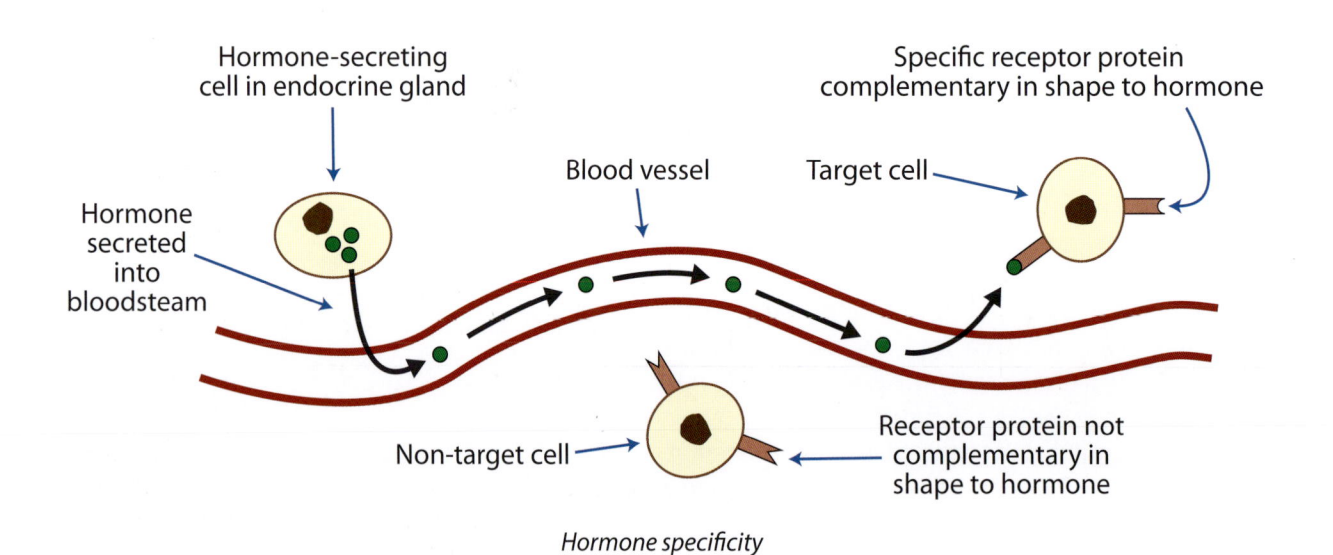

Hormone specificity

2.4 HOMEOSTATIC MECHANISMS AND HOW THESE ARE MONITORED

The table below summarises the role of a number of hormones in body function.

Gland	Hormone(s) produced	Target organ	Effect of hormone(s)
Pineal gland	Melatonin	Hypothalamus	Regulates the biological clock.
Pituitary gland	Anti-diuretic hormone (ADH)	Kidneys	Increases reabsorption of water by the kidneys.
	Follicle stimulating hormone (FSH)	Ovaries	Stimulates egg development and oestrogen production.
		Testes	Stimulates production of sperm.
	Luteinising hormone (LH)	Ovaries	Stimulates egg release, production of oestrogen and progesterone.
		Testes	Stimulates production of testosterone.
	Thyroid-stimulating hormone (TSH)	Thyroid gland	Stimulates secretion of thyroxine.
Thyroid gland	Thyroxine	All tissues	Increases rate of metabolism.
Thymus gland	Thymosin	Lymph nodes	Promotes production and maturation of T-lymphocytes.
Adrenal gland	Adrenaline	Heart, liver, bronchioles, blood vessels	Increases heart rate, and rate and depth of breathing. Raises blood glucose level so more glucose is available for respiration. Causes blood vessels to contract to redirect blood toward major muscle groups, including the heart and lungs.
	Aldosterone	Kidneys	Increases sodium reabsorption.
Pancreas – islets of Langerhans	Insulin	Liver	Converts excess glucose to glycogen (lowers blood glucose level).
	Glucagon	Liver	Breakdown of glycogen to glucose (increases blood glucose level).
Ovaries (female)	Progesterone	Uterus	Maintains the lining of the uterus.
	Oestrogen	Ovaries, uterus, pituitary gland	Controls ovulation and the menstrual cycle. Stimulates production of LH and suppresses the production of FSH in the pituitary gland.
Testes (male)	Testosterone	Male reproductive organs	Controls puberty and sperm production.

Regulation and monitoring of blood glucose levels

Blood glucose levels are maintained by the hormones **insulin** and **glucagon**. These hormones are produced by structures called **islets of Langerhans** in the **pancreas**. These structures contain two types of cells:

- **α-cells**, which produce and secrete the hormone **glucagon**.
- **β-cells**, which produce and secrete the hormone **insulin**.

Insulin and blood glucose

After a **meal**, the blood glucose concentration **increases**, especially if the meal is rich in carbohydrates. When the blood glucose concentration increases above normal, this acts as a **stimulus** that is **detected** by **β-cells**. In response, β-cells increase the production and secretion of **insulin**. Insulin travels in the bloodstream and binds to insulin receptors on target cells in **liver**, **muscle and adipose** (fat) tissue.

The effects of insulin include:

- stimulating the uptake of glucose into cells all over the body.
- increasing the rate at which glucose is used by cells in respiration.
- increasing the rate at which glucose is converted to glycogen for storage in liver and muscle cells.
- increasing the rate at which glucose is converted to fat for storage.

These effects cause the blood glucose concentration to fall. As the blood glucose concentration returns to normal this is detected by β-cells, which respond by reducing insulin secretion.

The graph on page 34 shows how blood glucose concentration typically varies after eating a meal.

> **Tip:** Insulin **lowers** blood glucose concentration – it is not enough to say that it controls blood glucose concentration.

> **Tip:** The lowering of blood glucose level by secretion of insulin is an example of **negative feedback**. Remember, negative feedback occurs when there is a change in the normal level of the factor under control, causing a response, restoring the factor to the normal level (set point).

> In this case, the change in the normal value occurs after a meal is eaten, resulting in an increase in blood glucose concentration. The increase in blood glucose concentration is the **stimulus** and is **detected** by **receptors** called β-cells in the islets of Langerhans. β-cells act as an **effector**, producing and secreting insulin. This causes a **response** to occur that brings about a **corrective mechanism**, resulting in the lowering of blood glucose concentration to the **normal value**.

Glucagon and blood glucose

After a **meal** has been absorbed completely, and during **physical activity**, the blood glucose concentration may **decrease** below normal. This decrease in blood glucose concentration acts as a stimulus and is detected by **α-cells**. In response, α-cells increase the production and secretion of **glucagon**. Glucagon travels in the bloodstream and binds to glucagon receptors on target cells in the liver.

The effects of glucagon include:

- stimulating liver cells to break down glycogen to glucose, releasing it into the blood.
- speeding up the rate at which amino acids and other substances are converted to glucose.
- reducing the rate of respiration.

These effects cause the blood glucose concentration to increase.

Low blood glucose concentration triggers the release of the hormone **adrenaline** by the adrenal glands. One effect of adrenaline is to stimulate the conversion of glycogen and amino acids to glucose. As the blood glucose level returns to normal, this is detected by α-cells, which respond by reducing glucagon secretion. The production of adrenaline also decreases.

The flow chart on the next page summaries the control of blood glucose concentration by insulin and glucagon.

> **Tip:** Do not confuse glucagon and glycogen.
>
> Glucose is stored as glycogen.
>
> Glucagon is a hormone that causes the breakdown of glycogen back to glucose.
>
> ```
>                    Insulin
> Glucose  ⇌  Glycogen
>                   Glucagon
> ```

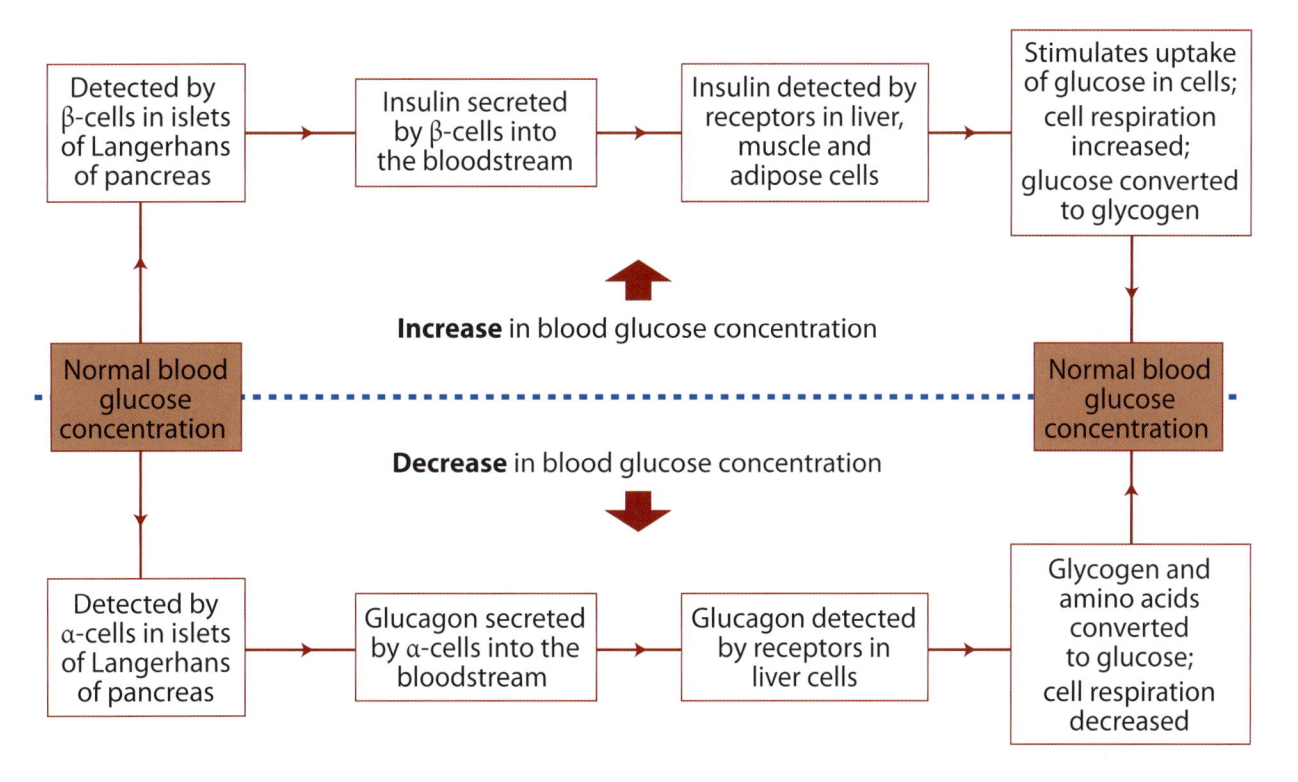

Control of blood glucose concentration by insulin and glucagon

Diabetes – when blood glucose regulation fails

Diabetes is a condition in which the body fails to regulate blood glucose levels.

- **Type 1** diabetes – results from a failure of insulin production by the β-cells where little or no insulin is produced.
- **Type 2** diabetes – is caused by insulin resistance. Target cells resist the effect of insulin and therefore build up a tolerance to insulin. When this happens, the pancreas starts to produce higher levels of insulin to bring the blood glucose concentration back down to normal. As the cells become increasingly more insulin resistant, the pancreas cannot continue to produce these high levels of insulin. The pancreas may become damaged and, as a result, little insulin is produced.

A person with diabetes has a higher baseline level of blood glucose concentration in comparison to a healthy person. After consuming a meal, a diabetic's blood glucose concentration peaks higher and the peak is delayed in comparison to a healthy person.

It takes longer for a diabetic's blood glucose concentration to decrease and it does not return to a healthy (non-diabetic) level.

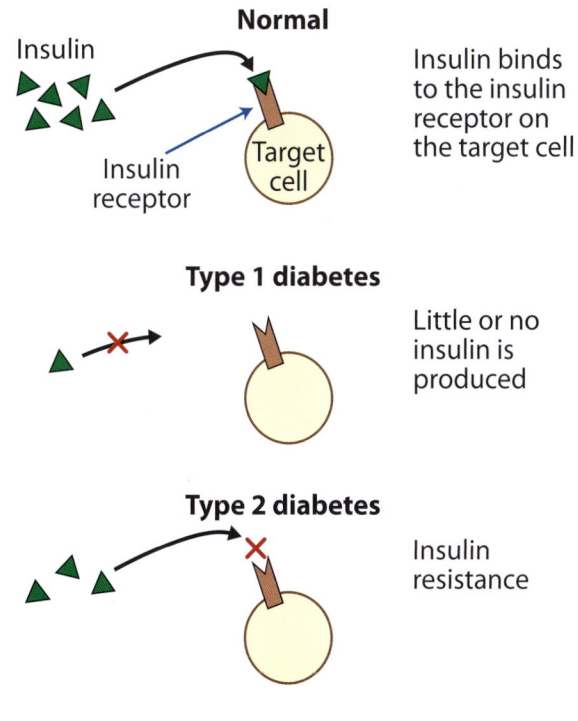

Insulin action, type 1 and type 2 diabetes

The graph below shows how blood glucose concentration typically varies after eating a meal in a healthy and diabetic person.

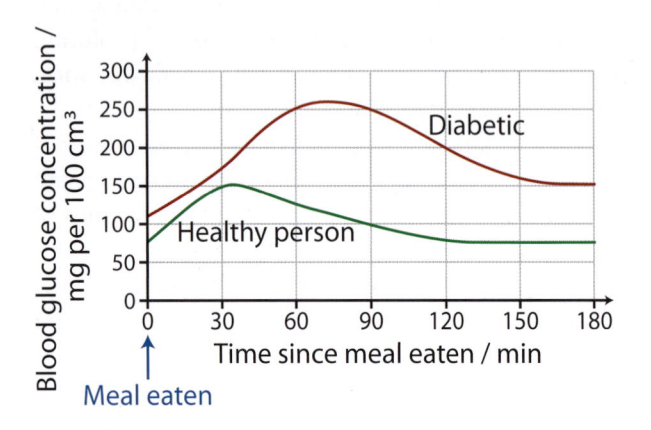

Blood glucose concentration in a healthy person and a diabetic person after a meal is consumed

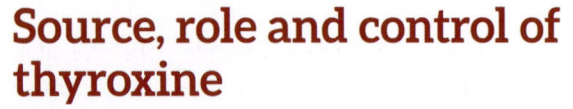

Source, role and control of thyroxine

Thyroxine is a hormone produced by the **thyroid gland**. The thyroid gland is an endocrine gland located in the neck. Thyroxine has a number of roles in the body, thyroxine:

- increases basal metabolic rate
- increases heart rate
- increases cardiac output
- increases ventilation rate
- potentiates (enhances) the effects of the catecholamines (i.e. increases sympathetic activity)
- potentiates (enhances) brain development
- thickens endometrium (lining of the uterus) in females
- increases metabolism of proteins and carbohydrates
- promotes growth

The regulation of thyroid hormone secretion depends on a **negative feedback** loop between the hypothalamus, pituitary gland and the thyroid gland.

The hypothalamus secretes thyroid-releasing hormone (**TRH**). This regulates the formation and secretion of thyroid-stimulating hormone (**TSH**) in the pituitary gland. TSH causes the thyroid gland to release thyroxine.

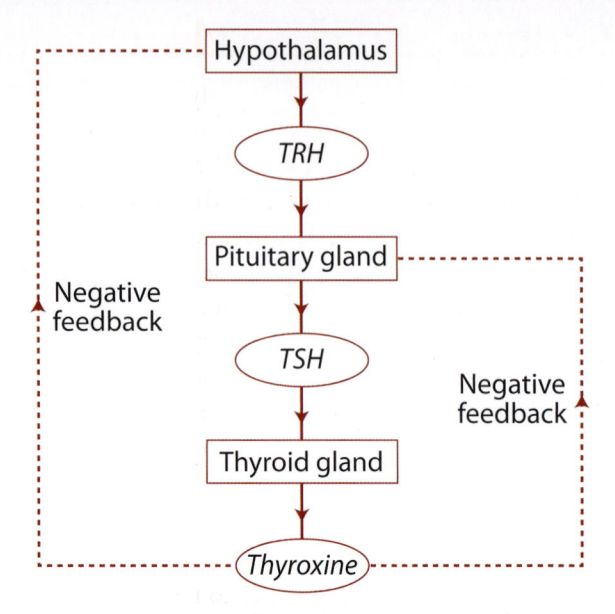

Control and regulation of thyroxine

When the concentration of thyroxine in the blood **rises above** normal, the pituitary gland secretes **less** TSH.

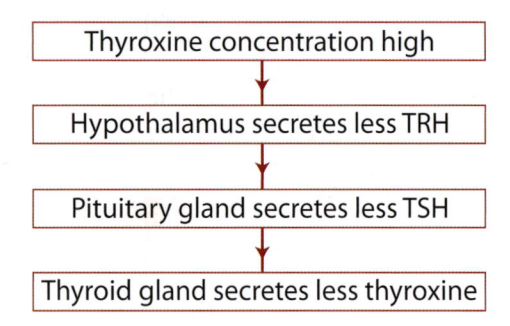

When the concentration of thyroxine **decreases**, the pituitary gland secretes **more** TSH.

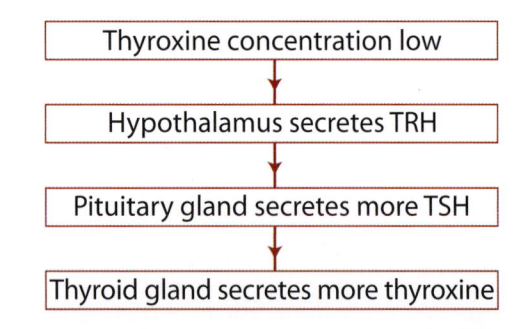

Tip: An **increase** in TRH or TSH will cause the thyroid gland to secrete **more** thyroxine.

Tip: A **decrease** in TRH or TSH will cause the thyroid gland to secrete **less** thyroxine.

Sodium and chloride ions

Sodium is one of the body's electrolytes. Electrolytes carry an electric charge when dissolved in body fluids such as blood. Sodium ions (Na^+) are the principal positive ion found in fluid surrounding cells. Sodium ions help maintain **water balance**, help the control of **blood pressure** and aid in **acid-base balance**, **muscle contraction** and **nerve conduction**.

Chloride ions (Cl^-) are the principal negative ions found in fluid surrounding cells. They help maintain **water balance** and **acid-base balance**. They are an important component of **hydrochloric acid** (HCl) in the stomach, which aids digestion.

Regulation of sodium

Several hormones work together to regulate sodium. The table below summarises the role of these hormones in the regulation of sodium.

Blood pH

The **pH** of a solution is a measure of the concentration of hydrogen ions (H^+) present. The higher the concentration of hydrogen ions, the more acidic the solution. The pH scale runs from 1–14. pH 7 is neutral, below pH 7 is acidic and above pH 7 is basic (alkaline).

An **acid** is a substance that increases the hydrogen ion concentration of a solution. A substance that reduces the hydrogen ion concentration of a solution is called a **base**. A base combines with H^+ ions, removing them from the solution, lowering acidity.

Blood is buffered to maintain a normal blood pH range between **pH 7.35–7.45**. Keeping the pH constant depends on controlling the relative concentrations of acid and base, the **acid-base balance**.

During normal metabolic processes, the body produces more acidic than basic waste products from:

- food consumed
- metabolism
- cellular respiration producing carbon dioxide

The body maintains blood pH balance in **three** ways:

1. **Buffer systems**
   Buffers are substances that keep the pH at a constant level. Buffers are able to minimise changes in pH by absorbing hydrogen ions from a solution when they are in excess and releasing hydrogen ions to a solution when they are in deficit.

Hormone	Secreted from	Effect of hormone
Aldosterone	Adrenal glands	Aldosterone increases sodium reabsorption in the kidneys. This prevents loss of sodium in urine.
		If sodium levels are above normal this will have a negative feedback effect and reduces the secretion of aldosterone from the adrenal glands. This results in more sodium being lost in urine, reducing blood sodium levels.
Antidiuretic hormone (ADH)	Pituitary gland	If sodium levels decrease, osmoreceptors in the hypothalamus are stimulated and cause the release of ADH from the pituitary gland.
		ADH acts on the kidneys, increasing the permeability of collecting ducts to water, therefore increasing water reabsorption. This increase in water reabsorption reduces the sodium concentration of body fluids and increases the sodium concentration in urine.
Atrial natriuretic peptide (ANP)	Atrium of the heart	ANP acts on the kidneys to promote sodium excretion. Sodium is excreted in the urine.
		ANP inhibits aldosterone secretion.

The role of hormones in the regulation of sodium

Buffer systems include:

- **Bicarbonate** (HCO_3) and **carbonic acid** (H_2CO_3), which can absorb or release H^+.

$$HCO_3^- + H^+ \longleftrightarrow H_2CO_3 \longleftrightarrow CO_2 + H_2O$$

- **Phosphates** in the blood.
- **Proteins** including **haemoglobin**. Proteins have amino groups (–NH_2) and carboxyl groups (–COOH) which can act as H^+ acceptors and H^+ donors respectively.

2. **Respiratory mechanisms**

During strenuous exercise, muscles produce carbon dioxide (CO_2) and H^+ as a result of increased metabolism. If the amounts of H^+ and CO_2 exceed the capacity of buffers to effectively control the blood pH, the lungs remove excess CO_2 from the blood.

Chemoreceptors are cells that are sensitive to changes in the presence and concentration of specific chemicals in the blood. Some are able to **detect** very small **changes in pH**. There are chemoreceptors in the aorta and the carotid artery. If a drop in pH (more acidic pH) is detected, impulses are sent to the respiratory centre of the brain. The respiratory centre sends more frequent nerve impulses to the diaphragm and the intercostal muscles. As a result, **breathing becomes faster and deeper**. As the lungs remove carbon dioxide, the hydrogen ion concentration in the blood and other body fluids decreases, and homeostasis is re-established.

3. **Kidney excretion**

The kidneys are able to affect blood pH by excreting excess acids or bases. The kidneys reabsorb hydrogen-carbonate ions and actively expel hydrogen ions which, after being buffered, are excreted in the urine.

Monitoring blood pH

It is vital that blood pH is monitored. Changes from normal blood pH (**7.35–7.45**) can result in serious health problems and potentially death.

Blood pH can be monitored in a clinical setting by obtaining an arterial blood sample. The test is commonly known as a blood gas analysis or **arterial blood gas (ABG) test**. An ABG test measures the amount of oxygen dissolved in the blood (PO_2) and the amount of carbon dioxide dissolved in the blood (PCO_2). It also measures the body's acid-base (pH) level.

Arterial blood can be obtained from an artery in a patient's wrist, arm or groin using a needle.

Acidosis and alkadosis

Acidosis occurs when blood pH falls **below 7.35**, indicating an increase in hydrogen ion concentration. **Alkalosis** occurs when blood pH rises **above 7.45**, indicating a reduction in hydrogen ion concentration.

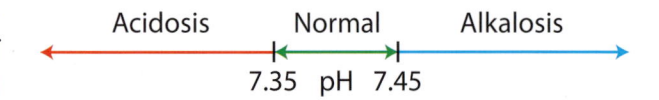

Acidosis   Normal   Alkalosis

7.35   pH   7.45

Acid-base disorders are divided into two broad categories – **respiratory** and **metabolic**. Those that affect breathing and cause changes in carbon dioxide concentration are called respiratory acidosis (low pH) or respiratory alkalosis (high pH).

The table below summarises the main causes of **respiratory** acidosis and alkalosis.

Main causes of respiratory acidosis	Main causes of respiratory alkalosis
Lung disease: e.g. chronic obstructive pulmonary disease (COPD), asthma or pneumonia	Hyperventilation due to extreme anxiety, panic attacks, asthma attacks, stress etc.
Decreased breathing due to medicines that suppress breathing	Stroke
Respiratory muscle or nerve diseases	Pneumonia
	Severe infection or fever

Disorders that affect bicarbonate concentration are called metabolic acidosis (low pH) and metabolic alkalosis (high pH).

The table below summarises the main causes of **metabolic** acidosis and alkalosis.

Main causes of metabolic acidosis	Main causes of metabolic alkalosis
Diabetic ketoacidosis	Excessive vomiting
Severe diarrhoea	Overuse of diuretics
Lactic acidosis	Excessive intake of drugs that are alkaline

Oxygen saturation

Oxygen saturation (SpO_2) is the percentage of haemoglobin-bound oxygen compared to the total oxygen binding capacity of the haemoglobin. **Normal SpO_2% levels are 94–99%.**

One haemoglobin molecule can carry a maximum of four molecules of oxygen. If a haemoglobin molecule is carrying three molecules of oxygen then it is carrying $\frac{3}{4}$ or 75% of the maximum amount of oxygen it could carry.

SpO_2% levels of blood can be **monitored** using a **pulse oximeter**. It measures how well oxygen is being sent to parts of the body furthest from the heart, such as the arms and legs. A clip-like device called a probe is placed on a body part, such as a finger or an ear lobe. The probe uses light to measure how much oxygen is in the blood.

There are a number of factors that affect oxygen saturation including **blood pH** and **temperature**. An increase in blood pH and decrease in temperature cause a decrease in the saturation of oxygen. **Hypoxia** occurs when the body is deprived of adequate oxygen.

The following conditions may lead to reduced SpO_2% levels:

- **Cystic fibrosis** is a genetic condition. Affected individuals have more mucus in their respiratory pathway than is normally the case. This, and the fact that the build up of mucus makes these individuals more prone to respiratory infections, leads to reduced gas exchange.

- **Emphysema** is a lung condition common in heavy smokers. Irritation from tar in cigarette smoke breaks down the walls of the alveoli, causing them to merge, forming fewer, larger alveoli. This reduces the surface area, resulting in **less diffusion** of respiratory gases. The **reduction in oxygen** causes a person to become short of breath, so their breathing rate increases.

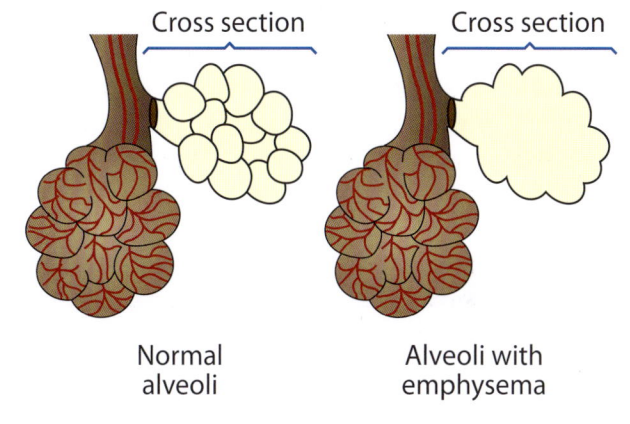

The effect of emphysema

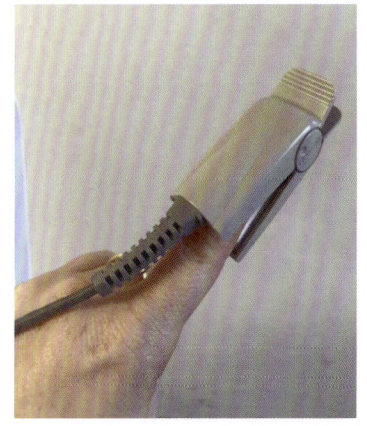

A pulse oximeter measuring SpO_2%
(Source: Jillian Neville)

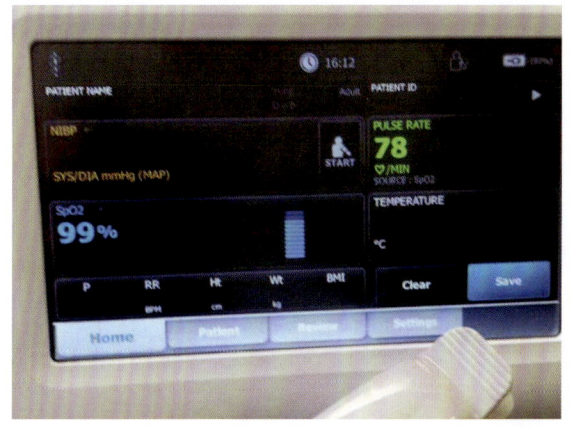

Monitor screen showing a patient's SpO_2 at 99%
(Source: Jillian Neville)

- **Pneumonia** is most commonly caused by a bacterial or viral **infection**. As the alveoli become infected they start to become inflamed and fill up with **fluid**. The increase in fluid reduces the process of gas exchange. This results in less oxygen reaching the blood stream and a rise in carbon dioxide in the blood. This causes a person to become short of breath.

Questions

1. (a) (i) Define the term homeostasis. [1]
      (ii) Give two factors controlled by homeostasis. [2]
   (b) Describe the role of the hormone adrenaline in body function. [2]
   [5 marks]

2. (a) (i) Name the cells that produce insulin. [1]
      (ii) Describe and explain the effect of insulin on blood glucose concentration. [3]
      (iii) Describe and explain the effect of glucagon on blood glucose concentration. [3]
   [7 marks]

3. The thyroid gland secretes the hormone thyroxine.
   (a) (i) State two roles of thyroxine in the body. [2]

   The flow chart shows how the body controls the level of thyroxine in the blood.

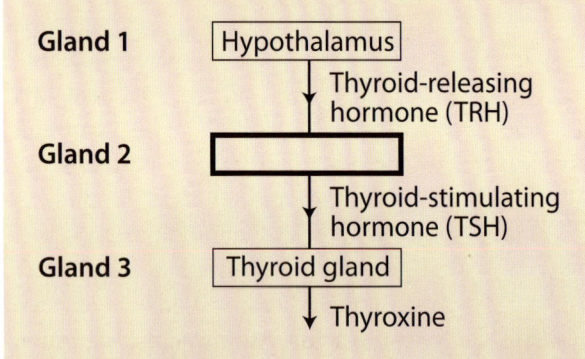

   Gland 1 — Hypothalamus
   ↓ Thyroid-releasing hormone (TRH)
   Gland 2 — [ ]
   ↓ Thyroid-stimulating hormone (TSH)
   Gland 3 — Thyroid gland
   ↓ Thyroxine

   (ii) Complete the flow chart by identifying **Gland 2**. [1]

   (b) State what will happen to the release of thyroxine if the secretion of:
      (i) TSH increases. [1]
      (ii) TRH decreases. [1]
   [4 marks]

4. A 65-year-old woman suffers from emphysema. The woman visits her doctor who measures her oxygen saturation.
   (i) Give the normal range for oxygen saturation of the blood.

   _____ to _____% [1]

   (ii) Describe how the doctor would measure the oxygen saturation of the woman's blood [1]
   (iii) Describe and explain the effect of emphysema on breathing rate in comparison to a healthy person. [2]
   [4 marks]

2.5 NUTRITION AND PHYSICAL EXERCISE IN MAINTAINING GOOD HEALTH

Students should be able to:

2.5.1 demonstrate an understanding of the importance of a balanced diet and regular physical exercise in helping to maintain good health;

2.5.2 describe the composition of a balanced, healthy diet for an average person, including the proportions of different food groups;

2.5.3 describe the short-term and long-term benefits of a balanced, healthy diet;

2.5.4 demonstrate an understanding that body mass is gained or lost when the energy content of food taken in is more or less than the amount of energy expended by the body, how food intake and physical activity influence body mass, and the effects of being overweight and of obesity on short-, medium- and long-term health;

2.5.5 collect, analyse and compare the composition of the diets of three or more individuals with a similar gender and age profile, critically evaluating their diets and classifying these as healthy or unhealthy;

2.5.6 compare the different nutritional and energy needs of babies, infants, young adults, pregnant women, adults and older people;

2.5.7 illustrate how a diet may need to be modified to suit the needs of specialist groups, for example diabetics, the overweight and obese, and older people;

2.5.8 describe the source, regulation and function of cholesterol, sodium, calcium, iron, and vitamins B, C, D and E;

2.5.9 summarise the monitoring of normal cholesterol levels (4.0–6.5 mmol/L) and the health effects of persistently high or low cholesterol;

2.5.10 explain how blood levels of iron, sodium and calcium are measured and monitored, the effects of deficiencies on health, and how these deficiencies may be rectified;

2.5.11 state normal levels of vitamins B, C, D and E, how these are monitored, the effects of deficiencies on health, and how these deficiencies may be rectified;

2.5.12 investigate current UK alcohol intake recommendations and the short-term and long-term health effects of alcohol consumption, including both positive (low-moderate consumption) and negative effects; and

2.5.13 evaluate short-term and long-term positive effects of regular physical exercise on general health, as well as cardiovascular and respiratory health.

A balanced diet

Food is essential for life. The human body needs energy for growth and activity.

A **balanced diet** should provide the correct amounts of **each** food group. This includes nutrient-dense foods to meet the body's energy needs and the correct nutrients to maintain health.

The Eatwell Guide (see next page) shows the different types of foods and drinks we should consume and the proportions for a healthy, balanced diet.

It divides the foods we eat and drink into five main food groups:

1. Potatoes, bread, rice, pasta and other starchy carbohydrates
2. Fruit and vegetables
3. Beans, pulses, fish, eggs, meat and other proteins
4. Dairy and alternatives
5. Oil and spreads

Macronutrients and micronutrients

There are five main groups of nutrients: protein, carbohydrate, fat, vitamins and minerals. **Macronutrients** include protein, carbohydrate and fat, and are required in much larger amounts. **Micronutrients** include vitamins and minerals, and are required in smaller amounts (see pages 43–47).

Proteins are needed for growth and repair of body tissues. Proteins are composed of **amino acids**. Amino acids made by the body are called non-essential or **dispensable** amino acids. Amino acids that cannot be made by the body are called essential or **indispensable** amino acids, and must be provided by diet. Sources of protein include beans, pulses, fish, eggs and meat.

Carbohydrates provide **energy**. Sources of carbohydrates include potatoes, bread, rice and pasta. **Fibre** is an indigestible form of carbohydrate. Fibre helps to prevent constipation and lower cholesterol levels. A diet high in fibre is associated with a lower risk of heart disease, stroke, type 2 diabetes and bowel cancer. Whole grain products, fruit and vegetables all contain high amounts of fibre.

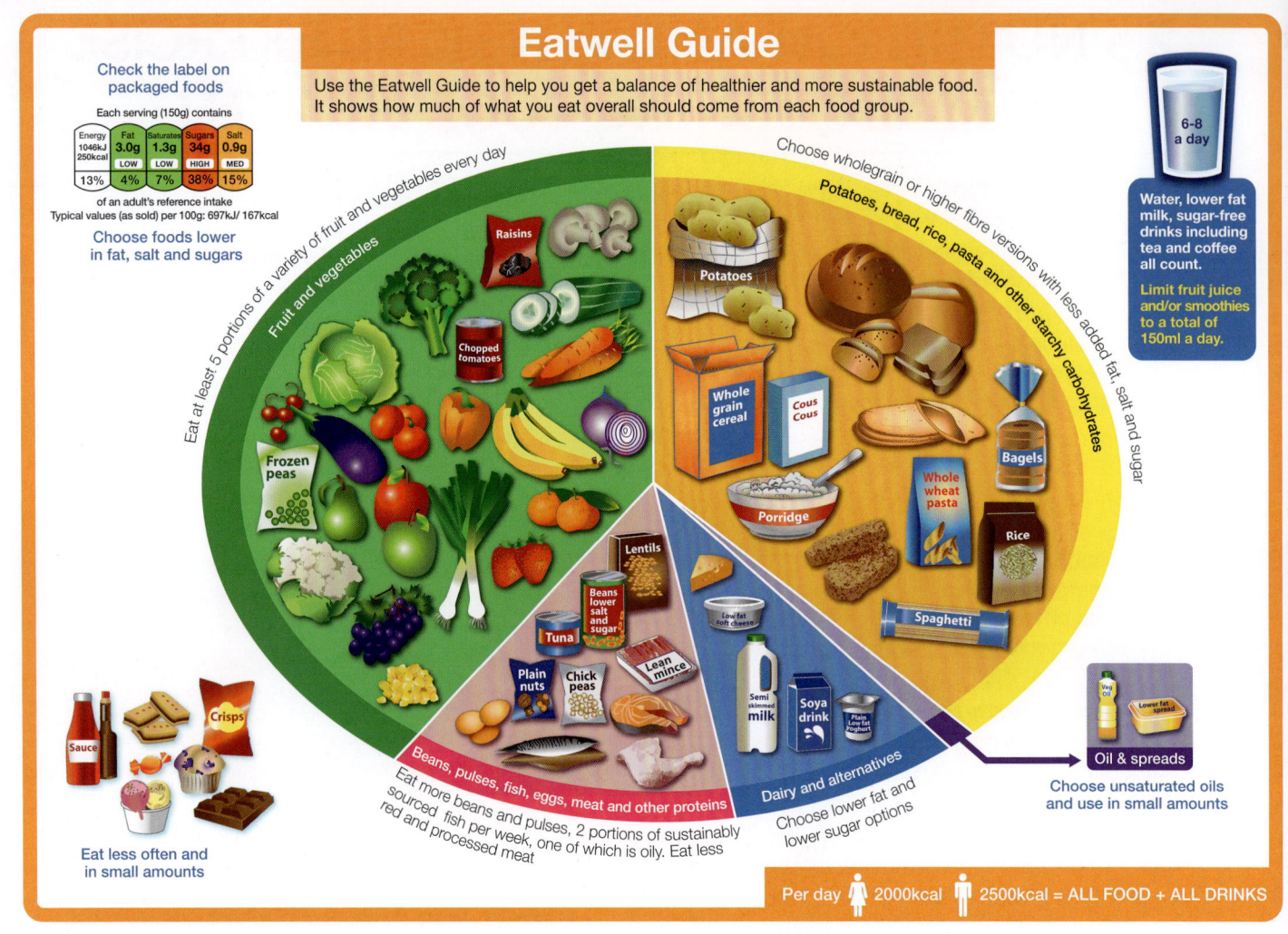

Fats are a source of **energy** and are an essential component of all **cell membranes**. Fats help the body absorb vitamins A, D and E. Fats can be **saturated** or **unsaturated**. Most saturated fats come from animal sources (including red meat) and dairy products (such as butter and cheese), and are found in biscuits, cakes and pastries. Unsaturated fat sources include olive oil, rapeseed oil, almonds, avocado, salmon and sardines.

Reference Intakes (RIs)

Reference intakes (RIs) are shown on nutrition labels of packaged food. RIs are a guide to the amount of energy and key nutrients that can be eaten on a daily basis in order to maintain a healthy diet. The values are maximum amounts based on an average female adult.

RIs for energy and selected nutrients are shown in the table below.

RIs help show the contribution a product or portion size makes to daily intakes. The nutrition labels on food packaging usually state the percentage of the daily RIs each product or portion contains. Food labels are also often colour coded to show high (red), medium (amber) or low (green) amounts of each nutrient.

Energy or nutrient	Reference intake
Energy	8400 kJ/2000 kcal
Fat	70 g
Saturates	20 g
Carbohydrate	260 g
Total sugars	90 g
Protein	50 g
Salt	6 g

(Source: Data from 'Nutrition Requirements', British Nutrition Foundation, 2017)

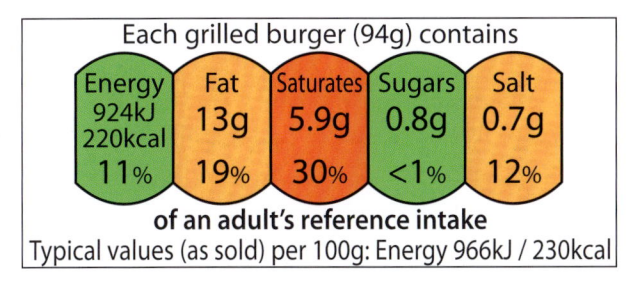

2.5 NUTRITION AND PHYSICAL EXERCISE IN MAINTAINING GOOD HEALTH

Each grilled burger (94g) contains

Energy	Fat	Saturates	Sugars	Salt
924kJ 220kcal	13g	5.9g	0.8g	0.7g
11%	19%	30%	<1%	12%

of an adult's reference intake
Typical values (as sold) per 100g: Energy 966kJ / 230kcal

Food label

(Source: 'Guide to creating a front of pack (FoP) nutrition label for pre-packed products sold through retail outlets', developed by the Department of Health, the Food Standards Agency, and devolved administrations in Scotland, Northern Ireland and Wales in collaboration with the British Retail Consortium. Contains public sector information licensed under the Open Government Licence v3.0.)

Age / years	EAR/kcal per day	
	Male	Female
1	765	717
4	1386	1291
10	2032	1936
16	2964	2414
35–44	2629	2103
55–64	2581	2079
75+	2294	1840

(Source: Data from 'Nutrition Requirements', British Nutrition Foundation, 2017)

Tip: You should be able to compare the different energy needs of babies, infants, young adults, pregnant women, adults and older people. There is more information on this on pages 42–43.

The food label above shows that each portion will provide 220 kcal, which is 11% of the reference intake for energy.

The food item contains 13 g of fat, which is 19% of the reference intake for fat. The amber colour indicates that the item contains a medium amount of fat.

The item will provide 30% of the reference intake for saturated fat and <1% of the reference intake for sugars. The red colour indicates that this item contains a high amount of saturated fat and the green colour indicates that it is low in sugar.

The item contains 0.7 g of salt, which is 12% of the daily reference intake for salt. The amber colour indicates that it contains a medium amount of salt. The recommended RI for salt is 6 g a day. A diet high in salt can cause high blood pressure (hypertension), increased risk of stroke, cardiovascular disease and kidney damage.

Energy requirements

Individuals vary in their energy requirements. Energy requirements depend on a range of factors including, age, gender, level of activity and state of health.

The following table shows the **estimated average requirements (EAR)** for energy.

Energy balance and body mass management

The key to maintaining a healthy body mass is to **balance** energy **intake** from food with energy **expenditure**. If the energy intake matches the energy expenditure there is no weight gain or loss.

Body mass is **gained** when the energy intake from food is more than the amount of energy expended by the body. The extra energy is stored by the body as fat. This energy imbalance can lead to a person becoming **overweight** or **obese**.

Being overweight or obese can increase a person's chances of developing high cholesterol, high blood pressure, type 2 diabetes, coronary heart disease (CHD), strokes, some types of cancer and mental health problems such as depression and anxiety. Being overweight or obese places more strain on hips and knees, which can lead to joint problems and osteoarthritis. Overweight people suffer more from gallbladder disease, sleep apnoea and breathing problems. Obesity during pregnancy increases the

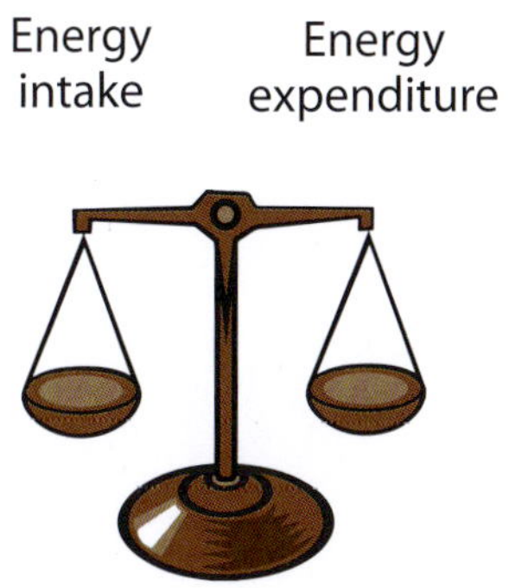

Weight maintenance — Energy intake / Energy expenditure

Weight gain — Energy intake / Energy expenditure

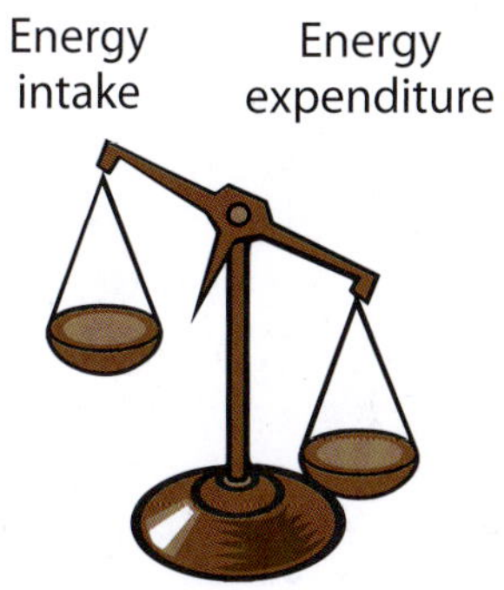

Weight loss — Energy intake / Energy expenditure

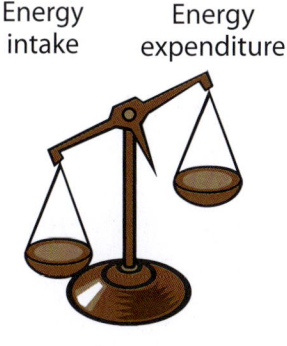

risk of pregnancy complications including gestational diabetes, pre-eclampsia and blood clots.

Body mass is **lost** when the energy intake from food is less than the amount of energy expended by the body. The fat stores in the body are used and body mass decreases. A decrease in energy intake and increase in energy expenditure through **additional physical exercise** causes a loss of body mass.

Changing nutritional needs

The nutritional needs of individuals changes with age.

Babies

During the early stages of life, babies undergo a period of rapid growth and development. Breast milk and formula milk contain all the nutrients required during this period. However, it is recommended that **breastfed** babies should be given a daily supplement of **vitamin D** as their bones are growing and developing very rapidly in these early years. Formula milk has vitamin D added during processing.

As babies grow, they have increased need for **energy, vitamins and minerals**. This cannot be met by a diet of milk alone. As a result, from 6 months of age, babies can be introduced to solid foods – this is called **weaning**. Babies should be introduced gradually to a wide variety of foods. It is important that the diet provided contains enough **iron** and **calcium** to meet the babies' needs for growth and development.

Infants

Infants have an increased need for **energy** to meet the demands of growth and physical activity. As children get older (4 years+) there is an increased need for **protein** alongside energy, particularly during periods of rapid growth and development. Infants should be given a 10 μg daily supplement of **vitamin D**.

Young adults

During adolescence, **energy** requirements continue to increase and protein requirements increase by approximately 50%, as teenagers experience an increase in their rate of growth. **Calcium** requirements increase dramatically from the age of 11 years. Calcium is important throughout childhood and adolescence for proper mineralisation of growing bone and to attain peak bone mass in adulthood. **Iron** requirements increase, particularly for adolescent females to make up for iron loss through menstruation.

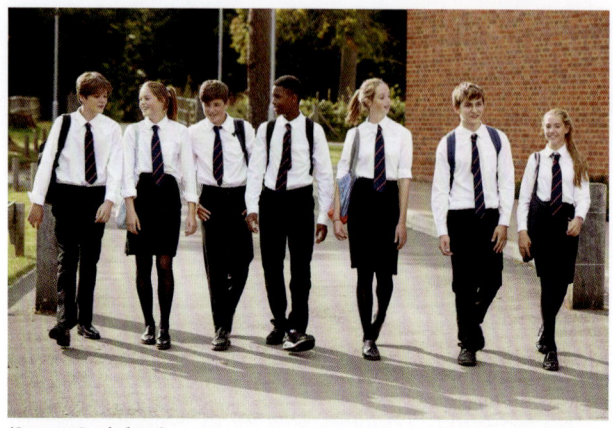

(Source: iStockphoto)

Tip: Peak bone mass is the stage at which bones have reached their maximum strength and density.

Pregnant women

During pregnancy, women require sufficient **energy** and **nutrients** from their diet for the developing foetus and the changes that take place in their bodies.

Before conception, and for the first 12 weeks of pregnancy, women are advised to take a 400 μg supplement of **folic acid**. Folic acid is important for the development of the spinal cord and can help to reduce the risk of neural tube birth defects, such as spina bifida, in unborn babies.

In all adults, including pregnant women, 10 μg of vitamin D is needed daily. Most commonly, a vitamin D deficiency occurs when the skin is not exposed to enough sunlight. In the UK, during the autumn and winter months there is no direct sunlight and the body's skin does not produce vitamin D. Vitamin D is especially important in foetal development and helps the baby grow strong bones.

Energy requirements for pregnant women increase by 200 kcal/day, but only in the final three months of pregnancy.

Pregnant women are advised to avoid any supplements containing vitamin A and foods rich in vitamin A (such as liver) as this could harm their babies.

Adults

During adulthood, it is important to maintain a healthy body mass by consuming a balanced diet and taking regular physical exercise. Energy requirements are lower for both men and women in comparison to young adults.

Older people

The nutritional needs of older adults are virtually unchanged from adults for both men and women. The main difference is that energy requirements decline due to a reduction in the basal metabolic rate and reduced levels of physical activity. However, many older people enjoy an active lifestyle. Meals should be nutrient dense rather than energy dense. Older people should ensure they include foods rich in **vitamin D** and **calcium** to maintain healthy bones. Some elderly people may not be outdoors often or may even be housebound. It is therefore recommended that they take a 10 μg daily supplement of vitamin D throughout the year.

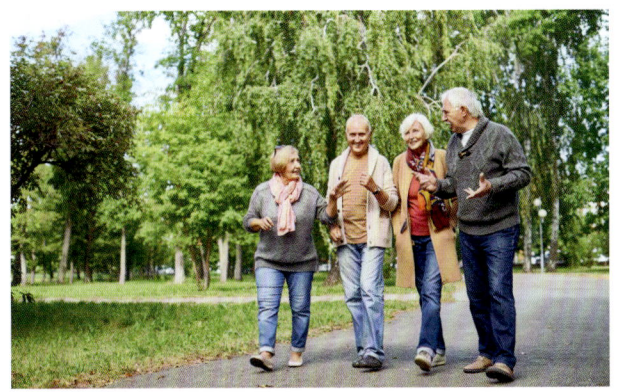

(Source: iStockphoto)

Diabetics

Diabetics should eat a **balanced diet** and follow the general dietary guidelines for healthy eating. Their diet should be high in starchy foods and low in sugary foods and drinks. Additionally, diabetics should eat **small meals** at **regular intervals** to help manage blood glucose levels. Diabetics should control their carbohydrate intake, and eat **complex carbohydrates**, which provide a slow release of glucose. As type 2 diabetes often occurs in people who are overweight, further lifestyle changes such as weight loss and increased physical exercise are advised.

> **Tip:** You should be able to collect, analyse and compare the composition of the diets of three or more individuals with a similar gender and age profile, critically evaluating their diets and classifying these as healthy or unhealthy.

Vitamins

Vitamins are **micronutrients**, as they are needed in small quantities to maintain good health.

Vitamins may be divided into **water-soluble** and **fat-soluble**. Water-soluble vitamins include **B group vitamins** and **vitamin C**. These vitamins dissolve in water and are easily destroyed or washed away during food storage and preparation, for example by boiling vegetables in water. These vitamins need to be replaced every day through the diet.

Fat-soluble vitamins include **vitamins D** and **E**. These vitamins are dissolved in fat before being carried in the bloodstream. The body does not need to replace these vitamins every day as fat-soluble vitamins are stored in the liver and fatty tissues when they are not being used.

The table on the following pages summarises the dietary sources, Reference Nutrient Intakes (RNIs), functions and deficiencies of vitamins.

Regulation and monitoring of vitamins

B group vitamins are initially regulated by intestinal absorption (bioavailability).

Vitamin C regulation is controlled by intestinal absorption (bioavailability), tissue transport, and renal excretion and reabsorption.

> **Tip:** Bioavailability refers to the amount of a nutrient that is absorbed from the diet into the body.

Vitamin D is a hormone. It is mostly produced by the skin in response to sunlight (90%) and obtained from diet (10%). **Vitamin D** remains in the body in an inactive form for 2–3 weeks. The inactive form of vitamin D can be activated by a specific enzyme. Vitamin D regulation is closely linked to calcium levels in the body. A fall in the level of calcium is detected by the parathyroid glands, which then produce parathyroid hormone. Parathyroid hormone increases the activity of the enzyme that produces the active form of vitamin D.

The **liver** is the master regulator of the body's **vitamin E** levels. It controls alpha-tocopherol (the most biologically active form of vitamin E) concentrations and also appears to be the main site of vitamin E metabolism and excretion.

The level of vitamins can be monitored through **blood tests**. A person's diet can be closely monitored to provide a balanced diet composed of the RNIs suitable for their age, gender and health status.

The table below summarises the dietary sources, RNIs, function and deficiencies of vitamins.

Vitamin	Dietary sources	Daily RNI* (male)	Daily RNI* (female)	Function of vitamin	Deficiency
Vitamin B1 (thiamin)	Fortified breakfast cereals, wholegrain breads, liver, potatoes, peas and eggs.	1.0 mg	0.8 mg	• Helps the release of energy from carbohydrates, fats and proteins. • Required for functioning and maintenance of nerves.	Vitamin B1 deficiency can cause **Beriberi**, a disease that affects the nervous system.
Vitamin B2 (riboflavin)	Fortified breakfast cereals, eggs, milk and spinach.	1.3 mg	1.1 mg	• Helps the release of energy from carbohydrates, fats and proteins. • Required for the development and function of the skin, lining of the digestive tract and red blood cells.	Vitamin B2 deficiency (**ariboflavinosis**) can cause skin lesions, such as cracks at the corners of the mouth.
Vitamin B3 (niacin)	Meat, wheat flour, eggs, fish and milk.	16.5 mg	13.2 mg	• Helps the release of energy from carbohydrates, fats and proteins. • Required for healthy skin and the function of the nervous system.	Vitamin B3 deficiency can result in a disease called **pellagra**, which can cause vomiting, diarrhoea, depression and the skin to become inflamed.
Vitamin B6 (pyridoxine)	Chicken, fish, milk, eggs, wholegrain cereals and vegetables.	1.4 mg	1.2 mg	• Essential for the formation of haemoglobin. • Important in amino acid metabolism.	Vitamin B6 deficiency can cause tiredness, numbness and tingling of the hands and feet.
Folate	Spinach, kale, broccoli, beans, legumes and fortified breakfast cereals.	200 µg	200 µg	• Folate is essential for the formation of red blood cells. • Important for the development of the spinal cord in unborn babies.	Folate deficiency can lead to folate deficient **anaemia**. Folate is important during pregnancy to reduce the risk of central neural tube defects, such as spina bifida, in unborn babies.
Vitamin B12 (cobalamin)	Meat, salmon, milk, eggs, cheese and fortified breakfast cereals.	1.5 µg	1.5 µg	• Essential in metabolism, manufacture of red blood cells, maintenance of the nervous system and metabolism of folic acid.	Vitamin B12 deficiency can lead to B12 deficient **anaemia** and other symptoms, including extreme tiredness and a lack of energy.

2.5 NUTRITION AND PHYSICAL EXERCISE IN MAINTAINING GOOD HEALTH

Vitamin	Dietary sources	Daily RNI* (male)	Daily RNI* (female)	Function of vitamin	Deficiency
Vitamin C (ascorbic acid)	Fruit and vegetables – including citrus fruits (e.g. oranges, lemons and limes), green and red peppers, tomatoes, broccoli and potatoes.	40 mg	40 mg	• Essential for the maintenance of healthy skin, blood vessels, bones and cartilage. • Required for the formation of collagen and absorption of iron. • Acts as an antioxidant.	Vitamin C deficiency can cause bleeding gums, wounds to heal slowly, skin to bruise easily or develop red or blue spots. Vitamin C helps to prevent the deficiency disease **scurvy**, which causes degeneration of skin, teeth and blood vessels.
Vitamin D	Oily fish, liver, milk and eggs.	10 µg	10 µg	• Aids in absorption and use of calcium and phosphate. • Promotes bone growth.	Vitamin D deficiency can result in weak bones. **Rickets** is a deficiency of vitamin D that occurs in children and is characterised by the development of bow-shaped legs, due to soft and weakened bones. In adults, vitamin D deficiency can lead to an adult version of the disease called **osteomalacia**, with a progressive softening of the bones. Osteomalacia can cause bones to fracture easily and severe bone pain in the back, pelvis, legs and ribs.
Vitamin E (tocopherols)	Plant oils (e.g. olive oil and soybean oil), eggs, prawns, spinach, broccoli, nuts and seeds.	4 mg	3 mg	• Acts as an antioxidant. • Required to maintain a healthy immune system. • Aids in the formation of red blood cells.	Vitamin E deficiency is very rare in a healthy person and is normally linked to a disorder that impairs fat absorption. A vitamin E deficiency can cause nerve and muscle damage, and a weakened immune system.

* Reference Nutrient Intakes (RNIs) are an estimate of the amount that should meet the needs of most people. RNIs of vitamins for adult males and females (19–64 years) are shown in the table.

(Source: RNI data from 'Government Dietary Recommendations', Public Health England, © Crown copyright 2016. Contains public sector information licensed under the Open Government Licence v3.0.)

Minerals

Minerals are inorganic nutrients, usually required by the body in small amounts. The table below summarises minerals' dietary sources, RNIs, function, deficiencies and the treatment of mineral deficiencies.

Mineral	Dietary sources	Daily RNI* (male)	Daily RNI* (female)	Function of mineral	Deficiency	Treatment of deficiency
Iron	Red meat, liver, eggs, spinach, broccoli, fortified breakfast cereals, legumes, beans, nuts and fish.	8.7 mg	14.8 mg	• Required for the formation of haemoglobin in red blood cells. • Required for normal energy metabolism and the metabolism of drugs and foreign substances that need to be removed from the body. • Required by the immune system for normal function.	A deficiency can result in **anaemia**. Tiredness, lack of energy, headaches, shortness of breath and pale skin.	Treatment focuses on the cause of anaemia. Patients may be prescribed daily iron supplements alongside vitamin C supplements to enhance iron absorption.
Sodium	Table salt and processed foods.	2.4 g	2.4 g	• Helps maintain acid-base balance, water balance, electrolyte balance, nerve transmission and muscle contraction.	A deficiency in sodium is rare. It can cause **hyponatraemia** resulting in headaches, vomiting, muscle cramps and seizures.	Treatment focuses on the cause of hyponatraemia. Patients may be treated with intravenous saline solution.
Calcium	Milk, cheese and other dairy foods, broccoli, cabbage, tofu, soya beans, sardines and white bread.	700 mg	700 mg	• Required for the formation of bones and teeth, blood clotting, nerve function and muscle contraction.	Deficiency disease is called **hypocalcaemia**. A deficiency can reduce bone mass: a contributory factor in the development of osteoporosis in later life. It can also cause nerve and muscle impairments, including pins and needles, spasms and an abnormal heartbeat.	Treatment may include calcium and vitamin D supplements or, in more severe cases, intravenous calcium gluconate.

* Reference Nutrient Intakes (RNIs) are an estimate of the amount that should meet the needs of most people. RNIs of vitamins for adult males and females (19–64 years) are shown in the table.

(Source: RNI data from 'Government Dietary Recommendations', Public Health England, © Crown copyright 2016. Contains public sector information licensed under the Open Government Licence v3.0.)

Regulation and monitoring of minerals

Iron in the body is mostly contained within haemoglobin in red blood cells and is also stored in the liver. Each day, a small amount of iron is lost; this is replaced as iron is absorbed from food by the duodenum.

Sodium is required in small amounts by the body. The regulation of sodium is covered in Chapter 2.4 (see page 35).

Calcium levels in the blood are tightly controlled. Blood calcium is regulated by a loss or gain of calcium from the kidneys, intestines or bones. The levels of calcium are controlled by three hormones:

1. **Parathyroid hormone (PTH)** is secreted in response to low blood calcium. It causes calcium to be released from bone, increases calcium reabsorption in the kidneys and increases the activity of the enzyme that produces the active form of vitamin D.
2. **Vitamin D** increases the uptake of calcium by the intestine.
3. **Calcitonin** is secreted in response to high blood calcium. It causes increased calcium excretion in the kidneys.

Iron, sodium and calcium blood levels are monitored through **blood tests**.

Cholesterol

Cholesterol is a fatty substance known as a lipid. Cholesterol is mainly made by the liver, but can also be found in some foods, including meat, fish, milk, eggs, cheese and butter.

Cholesterol is required to build and maintain cell membranes, make bile salts and steroid hormones, such as testosterone, oestrogen and progesterone.

Cholesterol is insoluble in blood so it is transported to cells and tissues by proteins. These complex molecules are called **lipoproteins**.

There are **two** types of lipoprotein:

- **High-density lipoprotein (HDL)** carries cholesterol away from cells to the liver. Here it is either broken down or passed out of the body as a waste product. HDL is referred to as 'good cholesterol'.
- **Low-density lipoprotein (LDL)** carries cholesterol to the cells that need it. If there is too much cholesterol for the cells to use, it can build up in the artery walls, leading to disease of the arteries. For this reason, LDL is referred to as 'bad cholesterol'.

A diet high in saturated fat can increase cholesterol levels, as well as other factors, including smoking, low levels of physical activity, obesity, diabetes, high blood pressure, high alcohol consumption and inherited conditions.

High levels of cholesterol (**hypercholesterolemia**) in the blood is strongly linked to **atherosclerosis**. This can cause blocked arteries due to the formation of **plaques** and **fatty deposits (atheroma)** on artery walls. Hypercholesterolemia has been linked to an increased risk of **coronary heart disease (CHD)**, heart attacks and **strokes**.

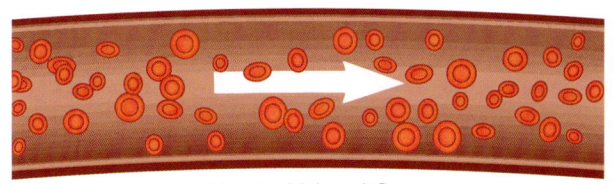

Normal blood flow

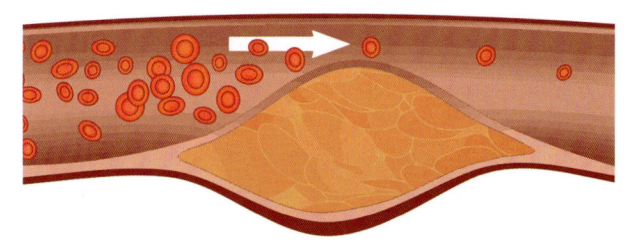

Plaque narrows artery

Atherosclerosis leading to blocked artery

Persistently **low** cholesterol (**hypocholesterolemia**) has been associated with an increased risk of cancer, stroke, depression and anxiety.

Regulation of cholesterol synthesis is carried out by the enzyme HMG-CoA reductase. The amount of cholesterol supplied in the diet will determine how much cholesterol is synthesised.

The normal level of total cholesterol in the blood should be within the range of **4.0–6.5 mmol/L** (millimoles per litre). Cholesterol can be **monitored** through blood tests. A blood sample is taken using a needle or a finger-prick test.

The effects of alcohol consumption

Current UK guidelines recommend that men and women should not drink more than 14 units of alcohol per week on a regular basis. If a person regularly drinks as much as 14 units per week, they should spread the units evenly over three or more days. It is also recommended to have several alcohol free days per week.

The guidelines state: "there is no justification for recommending drinking on health grounds, nor for starting drinking for health reasons".

The guidelines also advise anyone who is pregnant, or thinks they could become pregnant, that the safest approach is to not drink alcohol at all, to keep risks to the baby to a minimum. Drinking heavily during pregnancy can cause a baby to develop foetal alcohol syndrome (FAS).

(Source: Information from 'How to keep health risks from drinking alcohol to a low level, Government response to the public consultation', Department of Health, © Crown copyright 2016. Contains public sector information licensed under the Open Government Licence v3.0.)

Short-term effects of alcohol consumption

The short-term effects of alcohol can vary depending on a person's tolerance to alcohol and the number of units of alcohol consumed. Short-term negative effects **may** include:

- poor decision making
- slower reaction time
- lack of coordination
- speech begins to slur
- vision loses focus
- suffering from a 'hangover'
- headaches due to dehydration
- issues with digestion, leading to nausea, vomiting, diarrhoea and indigestion.
- injury or death from accidents and injuries, drowning, alcohol poisoning and self-harm related to alcohol.

Long term-effects of alcohol consumption

There are many long-term health **risks** associated with high alcohol consumption. These **may** include illness or death from:

- high blood pressure
- stroke
- liver disease
- different types of cancer
- mental health problems, including depression
- damage to the brain and nervous system
- pancreatitis
- sexual problems, such as impotence

Exercise and health

Regular physical exercise has many health benefits and lowers the risk of coronary heart disease (CHD), stroke, type 2 diabetes, cancer and early death.

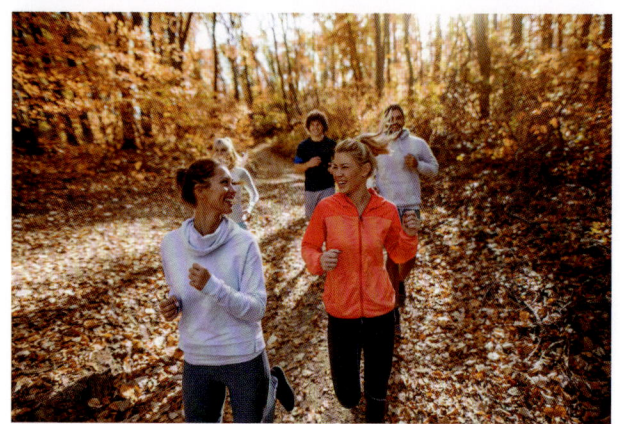

(Source: iStockphoto)

Exercise has many health benefits

Exercise can improve **social contact** and reduce the risk of depression, anxiety and stress, therefore improving **mental health**.

Exercise strengthens the ligaments, tendons, muscles and bones of the **musculoskeletal** system. Joints become more flexible, giving a greater range of movement and may lead to an increase in coordination. An increase in energy expenditure through additional physical exercise can help to achieve **weight maintenance**, reducing the risk of becoming **overweight** or **obese**.

2.5 NUTRITION AND PHYSICAL EXERCISE IN MAINTAINING GOOD HEALTH

Exercise and the cardiovascular system

Regular physical exercise benefits the **cardiovascular system**. Exercise **strengthens** the heart muscle, leading to an increased **cardiac output**. The cardiac output increases to deliver more blood, carrying oxygen and glucose to muscles for respiration.

> **Tip:** Cardiac output is the volume of blood pumped by the heart per minute.

Regular exercise **lowers** the **resting heart rate**. The time taken for the heart rate to return to normal is called the **recovery rate**. The recovery rate of a person who exercises regularly will usually be shorter than someone who does not exercise regularly. Regular physical exercise can reduce hypertension.

Exercise and the respiratory system

Exercise increases the **rate** and **depth** of breathing. Cells respire more during exercise – **more oxygen** is used and **more carbon dioxide** is produced. An increase in the rate and depth of breathing brings in a larger volume of air and increases the rate of gas exchange. Long-term exercise results in an increase in **lung capacity**.

> **Tip:** Lung capacity is the total volume of air that the lungs can hold.

Recommended physical activity for adults

The diagram below summaries the recommended physical activity that adults aged 19–64 should try to achieve each week to stay healthy.

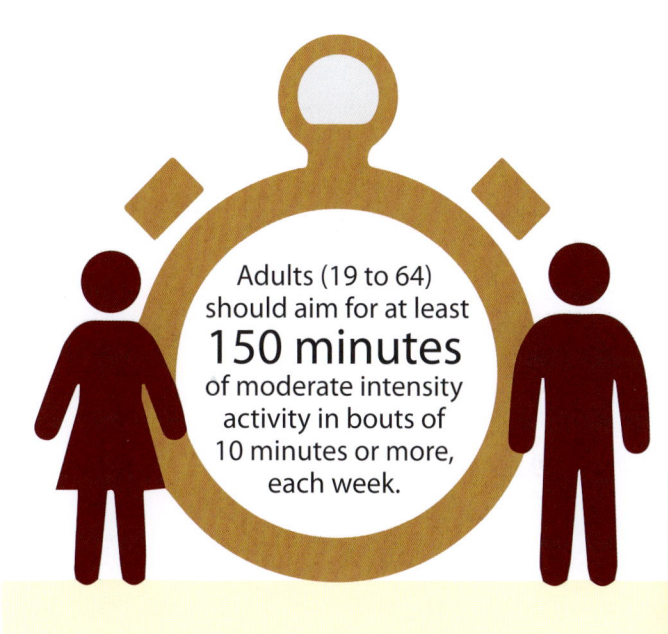

Adults (19 to 64) should aim for at least **150 minutes** of moderate intensity activity in bouts of 10 minutes or more, each week.

This can also be achieved by 75 minutes of vigorous activity across the week or a mixture of moderate and vigorous.

All adults should undertake muscle strengthening activity such as:

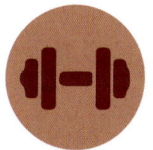

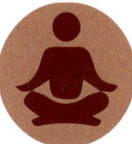

exercising with weights — yoga — or carrying heavy shopping

at least 2 days a week.

Minimise the amount of time spent sedentary (sitting) for extended periods.

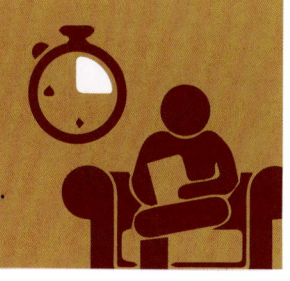

(Source: 'Health matters: getting every adult active every day', Public Health England, © Crown copyright 2016. Contains public sector information licensed under the Open Government Licence v3.0.)

Recommended physical activity for adults

Questions

1. (a) Give two food sources of calcium. [2]
   (b) Give two functions of calcium in the body. [2]
   (c) Give the name of the vitamin that helps the body to absorb calcium. [1]
   [5 marks]

2. (a) Describe and explain how an energy imbalance can contribute to obesity. [3]
   (b) (i) State two functions of vitamin B1 (thiamin) in the body. [2]
   (ii) Give two food sources of vitamin B1 (thiamin). [2]
   (iii) State the deficiency disease associated with vitamin B1 (thiamin). [1]
   [8 marks]

3. (a) Give two food sources of vitamin D. [2]
   (b) Describe a deficiency disease linked to lack of vitamin D. [1]
   (c) Explain why vitamin D supplements are recommended during pregnancy. [4]
   [7 marks]

4. (a) It was found that a man was consuming 8 units of alcohol per day on two days every week.
   (i) Give two pieces of advice to the man to reduce his health risks from drinking alcohol. [2]
   (ii) Give two harmful effects of alcohol on the man's long-term health. [2]
   (b) The table below shows the average daily amounts of energy, protein, vitamin C and iron the man is consuming, and the reference nutrient intakes (RNI).

	Energy /kcal	Protein/g	Vitamin C /mg	Iron/mg
Man	3000	40	25	5
RNI	2500	50	40	9

   (i) Comment on the man's average daily amounts of protein and vitamin C compared to the reference nutrient intake (RNI) figures. Make two recommendations of food sources that could improve the man's diet for protein and vitamin C. [4]
   (ii) Calculate the percentage of the RNI for iron the man is consuming. Give your answer to two decimal places. You are advised to show your working out. [2]
   [10 marks]

Unit AS 3: Aspects of Physical Chemistry in Industrial Processes

3.1 CHEMICAL CALCULATIONS

> **Students should be able to:**
>
> 3.1.1 use the chemical formula and relative atomic masses to calculate the relative formula mass of a substance, and the amount of a substance (moles) from its mass and vice versa; and
>
> 3.1.2 construct and use balanced symbol equations to calculate required quantities of reactants, theoretical yields of products, percentage yield from experimental data and theoretical yield.

Relative atomic mass (A_r) and relative formula mass (M_r)

The relative atomic mass is a measure of the mass of one atom of the element.

Relative atomic masses of all elements are given in the Periodic Table.

$$\boxed{\begin{array}{c}23\\ \text{Na}\\ 11\end{array}} \longleftarrow \text{relative atomic mass}$$

Relative atomic mass (A_r) is the **average** (weighted mean) **mass of an atom** of an element relative to one-twelfth of the mass of an atom of carbon-12.

The relative formula mass (M_r) is the sum of the relative atomic mass of all the atoms present in the formula of a substance.

Worked example
Calculate the relative formula mass of H_2SO_4.

Answer

M_r = (2 × relative atomic mass of H) + (1 × relative atomic mass of S) + (4 × relative atomic mass of O)

= (2 × 1) + (1 × 32) + (4 × 16)

= 98

Worked example
Calculate the relative formula mass of $Ca(NO_3)_2$.

> **Tip:** The number of atoms inside brackets is multiplied by the number outside – in this formula there are 1 × 2 = 2 nitrogen and 3 × 2 = 6 oxygen.

Answer

M_r = (1 × relative atomic mass of Ca) + (2 × relative atomic mass of N) + (6 × relative atomic mass of O)

= (1 × 40) + (2 × 14) + (6 × 16)

= 164

Worked example
Calculate the relative formula mass of $(NH_4)_2SO_4$.

Answer

M_r = (2 × relative atomic mass of N) + (8 × relative atomic mass of H) + (1 × relative atomic mass of S) + (4 × relative atomic mass of O)

= (2 × 14) + (8 × 1) + (1 × 32) + (4 × 16)

= 132

> **Tip:** Relative formula mass does not have units.

Atoms and molecules are so incredibly small that scientists needed to invent a convenient unit of measure for counting them. Chemists use a quantity called **amount of substance** for counting atoms and it is measured using a unit called the **mole** (abbreviated to mol).

Calculating moles

To calculate the number of moles of any substance use the equation:

$$\text{moles} = \frac{\text{mass (g)}}{M_r}$$

> **Tip:** If calculating the number of moles of an **element** use relative atomic mass (A_r) instead of relative formula mass:
>
> $$\text{moles} = \frac{\text{mass (g)}}{A_r}$$

Worked example
Calculate the number of moles in 19.6 g of H_2SO_4.

Answer
$M_r\, H_2SO_4 = (2 \times 1) + (1 \times 32) + (4 \times 16) = 98$

$$\text{number of moles} = \frac{\text{mass (g)}}{M_r} = \frac{19.6}{98} = 0.20 \text{ mol}$$

Worked example
Calculate the number of moles in 90 g of $Ca(OH)_2$.

Answer
$M_r\, Ca(OH)_2 = (1 \times 40) + (2 \times 16) + (2 \times 1) = 74$

$$\text{number of moles} = \frac{\text{mass (g)}}{M_r} = \frac{90}{74} = 1.2 \text{ mol}$$

> **Tip:** Your calculator gives this value as 1.216216216. It is best to round your number to one or two decimal places. In this case, one decimal place is used.

You can also rearrange this equation to calculate the mass of a given number of moles of a substance:

$$\text{mass (g)} = \text{moles} \times M_r$$

Worked example
Calculate the mass, in grams, of 0.5 moles of magnesium hydroxide ($Mg(OH)_2$).

Answer
$M_r\, Mg(OH)_2 = (1 \times 24) + (2 \times 16) + (2 \times 1) = 58$

$\text{mass} = \text{moles} \times M_r = 0.5 \times 58 = 29 \text{ g}$

> **Tip:** You may find a formula triangle, like the one below, useful. Simply cover up the quantity that you want to find to show the equation that you need to use. For example, to find moles, cover up moles and you are left with:
>
> $$\text{moles} = \frac{\text{mass}}{M_r}$$

Formula triangle

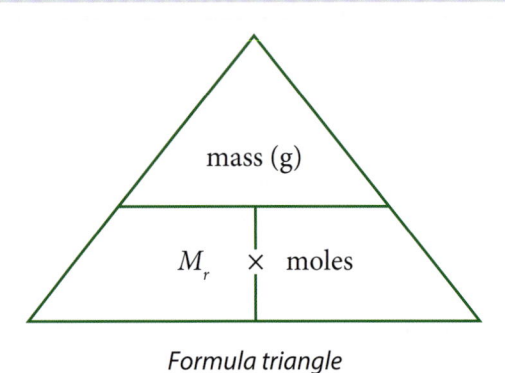

Converting units

When calculating masses in industry, grams is too small a unit for the quantities produced, and tonnes and kilograms must be used. However, to calculate number of moles the mass must always be in grams. If the mass is given in tonnes or kilograms, make sure you convert it to grams before using it in the equation.

1 tonne = 1000 kg
1 kg   = 1000 g

> To convert from tonnes to kilograms multiply by 1000 and from kilograms to grams, multiply by 1000.

3.1 CHEMICAL CALCULATIONS

Worked example
Calculate the number of moles present in 6.62 kg of lead nitrate, $Pb(NO_3)_2$.

Answer
Use the expression:

$$\text{moles} = \frac{\text{mass (g)}}{M_r}$$

First convert the mass from kg to g by multiplying by 1000:

$6.62 \times 1000 = 6620$ g

Calculate the M_r:
$M_r = (1 \times 207) + (2 \times 14) + (6 \times 16) = 331$

Calculate the number of moles:

$$\text{moles} = \frac{\text{mass (g)}}{M_r} = \frac{6620}{331} = 20 \text{ mol}$$

Worked example
How many moles of H_2SO_4 react with 0.4 moles of NaOH in the following reaction?

$$2NaOH + H_2SO_4 \rightarrow Na_2SO_4 + 2H_2O$$

Answer
Using the equation, write down the ratio between the two substances, and apply it to the 0.4 moles of NaOH:

$NaOH : H_2SO_4$
$\quad 2 : 1$
$\quad 0.4 : ?$

There is twice as much NaOH as H_2SO_4, so divide the number of moles of NaOH by 2:

$$0.4 : \frac{0.4}{2} = 0.2 \text{ mol } H_2SO_4$$

Molar ratios in equations

A **ratio** is a way to compare amounts of something. Ratios are written with a colon (:) between the numbers and usually only whole numbers are used.

In a balanced chemical equation, the substances are in ratio. The balancing numbers (the numbers in front of each species in the equation) give the ratio of moles that react together. For example:

$$2H_2 + O_2 \rightarrow 2H_2O$$

2 moles of H_2 react with 1 mole of O_2 to form 2 moles of H_2O.

The **ratio** is 2 moles H_2 : 1 mole O_2 : 2 moles H_2O

Or in the reaction:

$$2Al + 6HCl \rightarrow 2AlCl_3 + 3H_2$$

The ratio between aluminium and hydrogen is $2Al : 3H_2$.

The ratio between aluminium and hydrochloric acid is 2Al : 6HCl, which simplifies to 1Al : 3HCl.

The ratio can be used to calculate the number of moles that would react, or be produced, in any one equation.

Worked example
How many moles of aluminium (Al) are needed to produce 0.76 moles of aluminium oxide (Al_2O_3) in the following reaction?

$$4Al + 3O_2 \rightarrow 2Al_2O_3$$

Answer
Using the equation, write down the ratio between the two substances. In this case, simplify the ratio first and then apply it to the 0.76 moles of Al_2O_3.

$\quad Al : Al_2O_3$
$\quad\quad 4 : 2$
simplify: $2 : 1$
$\quad\quad ? : 0.76$

There are twice as many moles of aluminium as aluminium oxide, so multiply by 2:

$0.76 \times 2 = 1.52$ mol of Al

Calculating the mass of reactants and products

To calculate the mass of a reactant or product in a chemical reaction, the general method is:

- Underneath the balanced symbol equation, write down the **information** (mass) given in the question and circle the substance you need to find the mass of.
- Calculate the relative formula mass (M_r) or write down the relative atomic mass (A_r) of the substance you have information about and calculate the number of **moles**.
- Calculate the number of moles of the substance you need to find the mass of using the **ratio** from the balanced equation.
- Calculate the **mass** of the substance (using mass = moles × M_r).

Worked example
Calculate the mass of calcium carbonate that completely reacts with 3.65 g of HCl.

Answer
Write down the information (mass of HCl) and circle the substance you need to find the mass of ($CaCO_3$):

$\boxed{CaCO_3}$ + 2HCl → $CaCl_2$ + H_2O + CO_2

info: 3.65 g

moles: *Calculate the number of moles (of HCl).*
First, calculate the relative formula mass (of HCl):

M_r HCl = relative atomic mass of H + relative atomic mass of Cl
= 1 + 35.5
= 36.5

(Remember that the balancing numbers in the equation are not part of the formula and not included in M_r).

Then calculate the number of moles (of HCl):

moles of HCl = $\dfrac{mass}{M_r}$ = $\dfrac{3.65}{36.5}$ = 0.1

ratio: Use the ratio to calculate the number of moles (of $CaCO_3$):

HCl : $CaCO_3$
2 : 1
0.1 : ?

There are twice as many moles of HCl as $CaCO_3$ so divide by 2.

0.1 : $\dfrac{0.1}{2}$ = 0.05

mass: Calculate the mass (of $CaCO_3$).
First, calculate the **relative formula mass** of $CaCO_3$:

M_r $CaCO_3$ = (relative atomic mass of Ca) + (relative atomic mass of C) + (3 × relative atomic mass of O)
= 40 + 12 + (3 × 16)
= 100

Then calculate the mass (of $CaCO_3$):

mass of $CaCO_3$ = moles of $CaCO_3$ × M_r
= 0.05 × 100
= 5 g

Tip: Remember the order of calculation – **information, moles, ratio, mass**.

Worked example
Calculate the maximum mass of iron, in kg, produced when 400 g of iron oxide (Fe_2O_3) is heated with carbon monoxide.

Answer

Fe_2O_3 + 3CO → 2$\boxed{Fe}$ + 3CO_2

info: 400 g

moles: $Fe_2O_3 = \dfrac{mass}{M_r}$

M_r Fe_2O_3 = (2 × 56) + (3 × 16) = 160

moles = $\dfrac{400}{160}$ = 2.5

ratio: 1Fe_2O_3 : 2Fe
2.5 : ?
2.5 : 2 × 2.5 = 5

mass of Fe = moles × A_r
= 5 × 56
= 280 g

convert to kg: $\dfrac{280\ g}{1000}$ = 0.280 kg

Tip: The numbers in front of compounds in a chemical equation give the **ratio** of amounts that react – they **do not** affect the relative formula mass.

3.1 CHEMICAL CALCULATIONS

Percentage yield

The **theoretical yield** for a chemical reaction is the maximum mass of product that can be obtained. The mass of product that is actually produced in the laboratory is called the **actual yield** and is often less than the theoretical yield. The percentage yield of any reaction can be calculated using the equation:

$$\text{percentage yield} = \frac{\text{actual yield}}{\text{theoretical yield}} \times 100$$

> **Worked example**
> In a reaction, the theoretical yield of ammonia was 32 moles but the number of moles of ammonia actually produced was 24 moles. Calculate the percentage yield of ammonia.
>
> **Answer**
> $$\text{percentage yield} = \frac{\text{actual yield}}{\text{theoretical yield}} \times 100$$
> $$= \frac{24}{32} \times 100 = 75\%$$

The **percentage yield** is often less than 100%. This could be for many reasons:

1. Some of the product may have been lost during separation from the reaction mixture.
2. Side reactions may have occurred. This means that some of the reactants may have reacted in a different reaction to the desired one.
3. Some of the product may have turned back into reactants, as some reactions are reversible and do not go to completion.

In industrial processes it is important that the percentage yield achieved is as high as possible. A low percentage yield can mean a large waste of reactants and unnecessary expense. A high percentage yield means more product is formed from the available materials, reducing costs for the manufacturer, resulting in higher profit and/or the product selling at a lower cost to the consumer.

The theoretical yield for any reaction can be **worked out** using normal mole calculations and ratio as shown in the following example.

> **Worked example**
> (a) Calculate the theoretical yield of ammonium sulfate, in kg, when 1470 g of sulfuric acid completely react with ammonia.
> (b) In a reaction, a yield of 0.65 kg of ammonium sulfate was obtained. Use your answer to calculate the percentage yield. Give your answer to 1 decimal place.
>
> **Answer**
> (a) $2NH_3 + H_2SO_4 \rightarrow \underline{(NH_4)_2SO_4}$
>
> **info:** 1470 g
>
> $M_r \, H_2SO_4 = (2 \times 1) + (1 \times 32) + (4 \times 16)$
> $= 98$
>
> **moles:** $H_2SO_4 = \frac{\text{mass (g)}}{M_r} = \frac{1470 \text{ g}}{98} = 15 \text{ mol}$
>
> **ratio:** $H_2SO_4 : (NH_4)_2SO_4$
> $15 : ?$
> $15 : 15$
>
> $M_r (NH_4)_2SO_4 = (14 \times 2) + (1 \times 8) + (32) + (4 \times 16)$
> $= 132$
>
> **mass:** moles $\times M_r = 15 \times 132 = 1980$ g
>
> **theoretical yield:** $\frac{1980 \text{ g}}{1000} = 1.98$ kg
>
> (b) $\text{percentage yield} = 100 \times \frac{\text{actual yield}}{\text{theoretical yield}}$
>
> $= \frac{0.65}{1.98} \times 100 = 32.828\%$
>
> $= 32.8\%$ to 1 decimal place

> **Tip:** Percentage yields are also given as whole numbers.

Questions

1. Calculate the relative formula mass of:
   (a) NaCl [1]
   (b) NH_3 [1]
   (c) $Al(NO_3)_3$ [1]
   (d) $Pb(NO_3)_2$ [1]
   (e) $Ca(OH)_2$ [1]
   (f) $Ca(NO_3)_2$ [1]
   (g) $Fe_2(SO_4)_3$ [1]
   (h) $Cu(OH)_2$ [1] [8 marks]

2. Calculate the number of moles in:
   (a) 16 g of $Mg(OH)_2$ [2]
   (b) 50 g of $CaCO_3$ [2]
   (c) 54 g of $Al_2(SO_4)_3$ [2]
   (d) 5.6 g of $Ca(OH)_2$ [2] [8 marks]

3. Calculate the mass in grams of:
   (a) 0.3 mol of MgO [2]
   (b) 0.25 mol of $Ca(OH)_2$ [2]
   (c) 1.2 mol of Na_2CO_3 [2] [6 marks]

4. Calculate the number of moles present in:
   (a) 2.1 tonnes of iron (III) oxide (Fe_2O_3) [3]
   (b) 1.22 kg of magnesium nitrate $Mg(NO_3)_2$ [3]
   (c) 3.2 kg of calcium carbonate ($CaCO_3$) [3] [9 marks]

5. In the reaction $CaO + 3C \rightarrow CaC_2 + CO$:
   (a) how many moles of carbon are needed to completely react with 0.25 moles of CaO? [1]
   (b) how many moles of CO are produced when 1.2 moles of carbon react completely? [1] [2 marks]

6. 2.1 g of sodium hydrogen carbonate is heated until it completely decomposes and forms sodium carbonate, as shown in the equation below:
   $2NaHCO_3 \rightarrow Na_2CO_3 + CO_2 + H_2O$
   (a) Calculate the relative formula mass of $NaHCO_3$. [1]
   (b) Calculate the number of moles in 2.1 g of $NaHCO_3$. [1]
   (c) Calculate the number of moles of sodium carbonate produced. [1]
   (d) Calculate the mass of sodium carbonate produced. [2] [5 marks]

7. Calculate the mass of NO_2 obtained from complete decomposition of 33.1 g of lead nitrate. [3]
   $2Pb(NO_3)_2 \rightarrow 2PbO + 4NO_2 + O_2$ [3 marks]

8. Calculate the maximum mass of hydrochloric acid, in kg, required to produce 0.475 tonnes of magnesium chloride. [5]
   $Mg(OH)_2 + 2HCl \rightarrow MgCl_2 + 2H_2O$ [5 marks]

9. Calculate the percentage yield of NO if 6200 g of ammonia completely reacts with excess oxygen and produces 8 kg of NO. Give your answer to one decimal place. [6]
   $4NH_3 + 5O_2 \rightarrow 4NO + 6H_2O$ [6 marks]

10. Phenol (C_6H_5OH) is converted to trichlorophenol (TCP) ($C_6H_2Cl_3OH$) according to the equation below:
    $C_6H_5OH + 3Cl_2 \rightarrow C_6H_2Cl_3OH + 3HCl$
    (a) Calculate the maximum mass of TCP that can be produced from 23.5 g of phenol. Give your answer to one decimal place. [3]
    (b) If 38.1 g of TCP was actually produced in the reaction, calculate the percentage yield. [2] [5 marks]

3.2 VOLUMETRIC ANALYSIS

Students should be able to:

3.2.1 describe the techniques and procedures used to prepare a standard solution of the required concentration;

3.2.2 demonstrate an understanding of the techniques and procedures used when carrying out acid-base titrations involving strong acid/strong base, strong acid/weak base and weak acid/strong base (for example analysis of vinegar (ethanoic acid) or car battery acid (sulfuric acid));

3.2.3 select the correct indicator for each type of titration and recall the colour change of phenolphthalein and methyl orange at the end point;

3.2.4 select appropriate titration data, ignoring anomalies, to calculate mean titres;

3.2.5 calculate concentrations and volumes using titration data; and

3.2.6 employ the term molarity, M, and the units of concentration, for example mol dm^{-3}.

Concentration

Chemists can measure the concentration of a solution by considering the number of **moles** of solute that dissolve in **1 dm^3** of solution.

1 dm^3 is 1 decimetre cubed and it is a unit of volume.
1 dm^3 = 1000 cm^3 = 1 litre

Concentration is the number of moles of a solid that is dissolved in 1 dm^3 of solution.

The unit of concentration is **mol dm^{-3}**. For example, a solution that has a concentration of 0.2 mol dm^{-3} has 0.2 moles of solute dissolved in 1 dm^3 of solution.

To calculate concentration in mol dm^{-3}, the expression below can be used:

$$\text{concentration (mol dm}^{-3}\text{)} = \frac{\text{moles}}{\text{volume (dm}^3\text{)}}$$

Tip: You may wish to use a formula triangle like the one that follows to help you with your calculations. Cover up the quantity you want to find to show the equation you need to use.

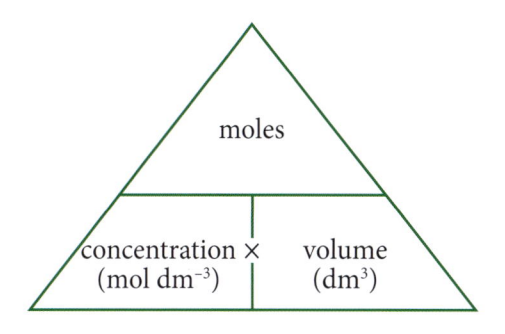

Formula triangle

If the volume is given in cm^3, it must be converted to dm^3 by dividing by 1000. If the volume in the question is given in cm^3, you may find it easier to use the equation:

$$\text{concentration (mol dm}^{-3}\text{)} = \frac{\text{moles} \times 1000}{\text{volume (cm}^3\text{)}}$$

Another word for concentration in mol dm^{-3} is **molarity**.

Molarity is the number of moles of a solid that is dissolved in 1 dm^3 of solution. The unit of molarity is **M**.

$$\text{molarity (M)} = \frac{\text{moles} \times 1000}{\text{volume (cm}^3\text{)}}$$

Tip: Molarity is the same as concentration – it is the number of moles in 1 dm^3.

Worked example
Find the concentration of each of the following solutions in mol dm^{-3}:

(a) 10 moles of solute dissolved in 5 dm^3.

Answer
$$\text{concentration (mol dm}^{-3}\text{)} = \frac{\text{moles}}{\text{volume (dm}^3\text{)}}$$
$$= \frac{10}{5}$$
$$= 2 \text{ mol dm}^{-3}$$

Worked example
(b) 0.60 moles of solute dissolved in 100 cm³.

Answer
$$\text{concentration (mol dm}^{-3}) = \frac{\text{moles} \times 1000}{\text{volume (cm}^3)}$$
$$= \frac{0.60 \times 1000}{100}$$
$$= 6 \text{ mol dm}^{-3}$$

Worked example
Calculate the molarity of a solution that contains 0.20 mol of solute dissolved in 50 cm³ of solution.

Answer
$$\text{molarity (M)} = \frac{\text{moles} \times 1000}{\text{volume (cm}^3)} = \frac{0.20 \times 1000}{50}$$
$$= 4 \text{ M}$$

It is also possible to work out the concentration of a solution if the mass of a solid, and the volume it is dissolved in, is given. To do this, you first need to work out the number of moles of the solid present using the equation:

$$\text{moles} = \frac{\text{mass (g)}}{\text{relative formula mass } (M_r)}$$

Worked example
Calculate the concentration of the solution formed when 49 g of H_2SO_4 is dissolved in 200 cm³.

Answer
First work out the number of moles of sulfuric acid in 49 g.
relative formula mass (M_r)
$= (2 \times 1) + (1 \times 32) + (4 \times 16) = 98$

$$\text{moles of } H_2SO_4 = \frac{\text{mass (g)}}{M_r} = \frac{49}{98} = 0.5$$

$$\text{concentration (mol dm}^{-3}) = \frac{\text{moles} \times 1000}{\text{volume (cm}^3)} = \frac{0.5 \times 1000}{200}$$
$$= 2.5 \text{ mol dm}^{-3}$$

Worked example
Calculate the molarity of a solution containing 54.75 g of HCl dissolved in 2000 cm³ of solution.

Answer
relative formula mass: $M_r = 1 + 35.5 = 36.5$

$$\text{moles of HCl} = \frac{\text{mass (g)}}{M_r} = \frac{54.75}{36.5} = 1.5 \text{ mol}$$

$$\text{molarity (M)} = \frac{\text{moles} \times 1000}{\text{volume (cm}^3)} = \frac{1.5 \times 1000}{2000}$$
$$= 0.75 \text{ M}$$

Preparing a standard solution

A standard solution is a solution for which the concentration is accurately known.

To prepare a standard solution, an accurately known mass must be dissolved in deionised water and the solution made up to an accurate volume using a volumetric flask.

The method to prepare a standard solution is:

- Weigh out an accurate mass of a solid (or liquid) in a clean, dry beaker using a top pan balance.
- Dissolve the solid in a small volume (50–100 cm³) of deionised water. Stir with a glass rod.
- Transfer the solution to a 250 cm³ (or other appropriately sized) volumetric flask.
- Rinse the beaker and glass rod with deionised water and add the rinsings into the volumetric flask.
- Make up to the mark by adding deionised water until the bottom of the meniscus is on the mark.
- Stopper the flask and invert to mix thoroughly.

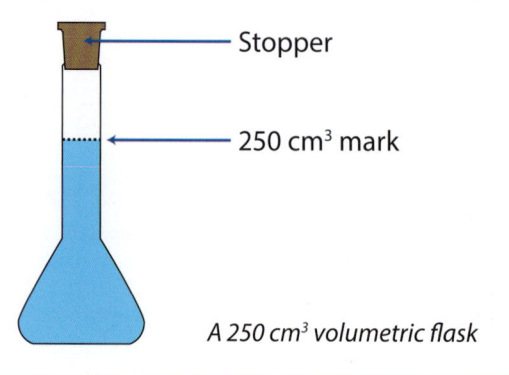

A 250 cm³ volumetric flask

Tip: A meniscus is the curved surface at the top of a column of liquid.

3.2 VOLUMETRIC ANALYSIS

Calculating the number of moles present in a solution

A useful rearrangement of the expression:

$$\text{concentration (mol dm}^{-3}) = \frac{\text{moles} \times 1000}{\text{volume (cm}^3)}$$

is:

$$\text{moles} = \frac{\text{volume (cm}^3) \times \text{conc (mol dm}^{-3})}{1000}$$

Similarly, if the volume is **given in dm³**, then an arrangement of:

$$\text{concentration (mol dm}^{-3}) = \frac{\text{moles}}{\text{volume (cm}^3)}$$

is:

moles = volume (dm³) × concentration (mol dm⁻³)

This expression can be used to calculate the number of moles present in a solution.

Worked example

Calculate the number of moles of solute in each of the following solutions:

(a) 15 dm³ of 0.50 mol dm⁻³ solution
(b) 25 cm³ of 1.2 mol dm⁻³ solution

Answer

(a) moles = volume (dm³) × conc (mol dm⁻³)
   = 15 × 0.50
   = 7.5 mol

(b) moles = $\frac{\text{volume (cm}^3) \times \text{conc (mol dm}^{-3})}{1000}$

   = $\frac{25 \times 1.2}{1000}$

   = 0.030 mol

Titrations

A titration is a very accurate experimental technique used to determine the volume of solutions, usually acid and alkali, that react together. This information can be used to find the concentration of a solution. Titrations are often used to find the concentration of acids or alkalis.

A **base** is a metal oxide or metal hydroxide that neutralises an acid to produce a salt and water. An **alkali** is a soluble base.

> **Tip:** A salt is the compound formed when some or all of the hydrogen ions of an acid are replaced by metal or ammonium ions.

The general reaction that occurs between an acid and a base during a titration is a neutralisation:

base + acid → salt + water

or more specifically:

alkali + acid → salt + water

Each acid produces a differently named salt. The following table shows the general names of salts formed by some acids.

Acid	Formula of acid	Salt
hydrochloric	HCl	chloride
sulfuric (car battery acid)	H_2SO_4	sulfate
nitric	HNO_3	nitrate
ethanoic acid (vinegar)	CH_3COOH	ethanoate

Below are some of the neutralisation reactions that you may carry out titrations for:

- sodium hydroxide + hydrochloric acid → sodium chloride + water
  $NaOH_{(aq)}$ + $HCl_{(aq)}$ → $NaCl_{(aq)}$ + $H_2O_{(l)}$

- potassium hydroxide + sulfuric acid → potassium sulfate + water
  $2KOH_{(aq)}$ + $H_2SO_{4(aq)}$ → $K_2SO_{4(aq)}$ + $H_2O_{(l)}$

- sodium hydroxide + nitric acid → sodium nitrate + water
  $NaOH_{(aq)}$ + $HNO_{3(aq)}$ → $NaNO_{3(aq)}$ + $H_2O_{(l)}$

- sodium hydroxide + ethanoic acid → sodium ethanoate + water
  $NaOH_{(aq)}$ + $CH_3COOH_{(aq)}$ → $CH_3COONa_{(aq)}$ + $H_2O_{(l)}$

- ammonia + sulfuric acid → ammonium sulfate
  $2NH_{3(aq)}$ + $H_2SO_{4(aq)}$ → $(NH_4)_2SO_{4(aq)}$

Titration apparatus

In a titration, a known volume of one solution is placed in a conical flask, using a pipette with safety filler, and a few drops of indicator are added. The other solution is added from the burette until the indicator changes colour, and the volume added is recorded. The standard solution is usually placed in the burette. A labelled diagram of the assembled apparatus set up for a titration is shown below.

> **Tip:** A measuring cylinder measures a solution only to the nearest cm^3 and so is not accurate enough to measure out volumes in titrations. A pipette, which is accurate to one decimal place, is used instead.

Choice of indicator

In a titration, the **end point** is where the indicator changes colour and the titration is stopped because the correct amount of acid and alkali have been added, and the reaction is over.

You need to learn the names and colour changes of the indicators shown in the table below.

Titration	Colour change	
	Methyl orange	Phenolphthalein
acid in conical flask alkali in burette	red to yellow	colourless to pink
alkali in conical flask acid in burette	yellow to red	pink to colourless

The indicator used depends on the strength of acid and alkali used in the titration. There are different strengths of acid and alkali. Strong acids have an approximate pH of 0–2 and weak acids have an approximate pH of 3–6. It is useful to know the common strong and weak acids shown in the table below.

Acid	Strength of acid	Formula
hydrochloric	strong	HCl
sulfuric acid (car battery acid)	strong	H_2SO_4
nitric acid	strong	HNO_3
ethanoic acid (vinegar)	weak	CH_3COOH

Strong alkalis have an approximate pH of 11–14 and weak alkalis have an approximate pH of 8–10. You should also learn the names and strengths of the alkalis shown in the table below.

Alkali	Strength of alkali	Formula
sodium hydroxide	strong	NaOH
potassium hydroxide	strong	KOH
ammonia	weak	NH_3
sodium carbonate	weak	Na_2CO_3

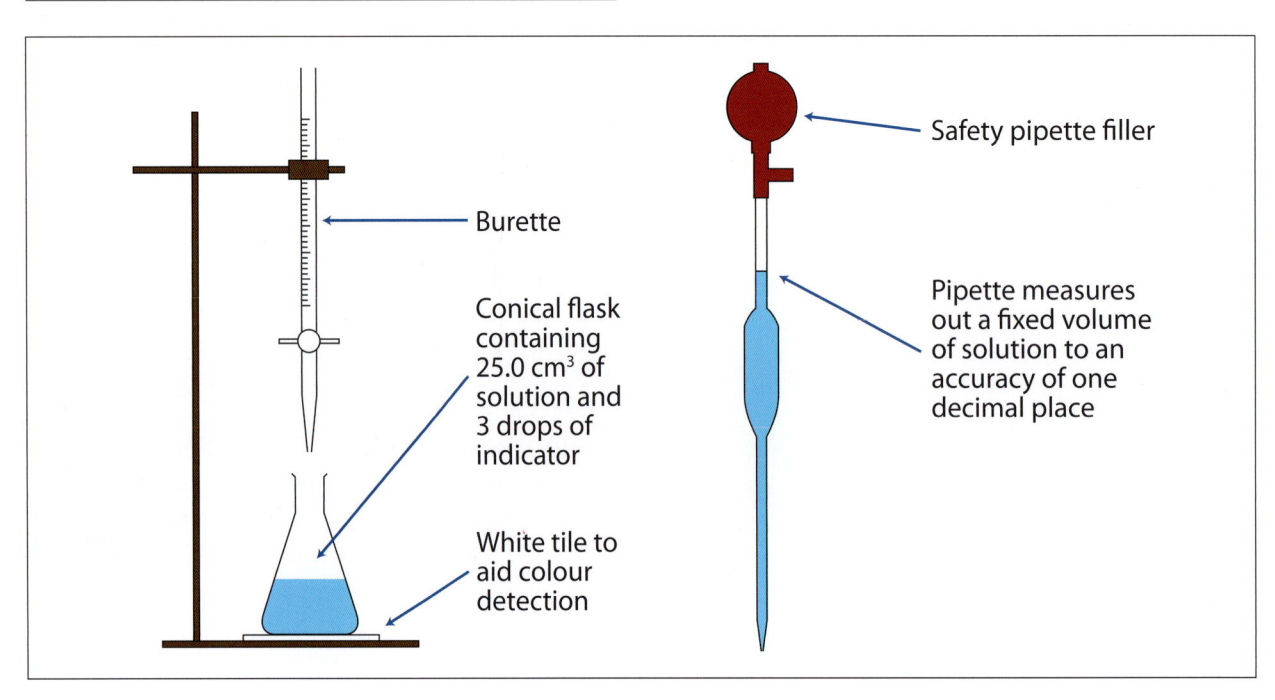

Titration apparatus

The table below shows the correct indicator to use for each type of titration.

Type of titration	Correct indicator	Example
strong acid, strong base	methyl orange or phenolphthalein	hydrochloric acid with sodium hydroxide
strong acid, weak base	methyl orange	sulfuric acid with ammonia
weak acid, strong base	phenolphthalein	ethanoic acid with sodium hydroxide

Tip: You need to learn this table.

Worked example
25.0 cm³ of sodium hydroxide solution was placed in a conical flask and titrated with ethanoic acid solution until the end point was reached. Explain which indicator could be used in this titration and state the colour change at the end point.

Answer
Sodium hydroxide is a strong alkali and ethanoic acid is a weak acid so the correct indicator to use in a strong alkali, weak acid titration is phenolphthalein. The sodium hydroxide is in the conical flask so the colour change is from pink to colourless.

Method of titration

1. Preparing the burette

- Rinse the burette with deionised water, followed by the solution it is to be filled with and discard the rinsings.
- Fill the burette with the solution.
- Make sure that the jet is filled and there are no air bubbles in the burette.
- Record the volume at the bottom of the meniscus at eye level to one decimal place – if two decimal places are used, the second decimal place must be 0 or 5.

2. Preparing and using the pipette

- Rinse the pipette with deionised water, followed by the solution to be transferred to the conical flask.
- Use a safety pipette filler and pipette to draw up the solution until the bottom of meniscus is on the line.
- Release the solution from the pipette into a conical flask.
- Touch the pipette on the surface of the liquid to remove the last drops in the pipette.

Tip: Never 'pour' from a pipette, it is best to use the words 'release' or 'expel'.

3. The method for carrying out a titration is:

- Use a pipette with a safety filler to measure out a volume of a solution (usually 25.0 cm³) and place in a conical flask.
- Add 2–3 drops of an indicator such as methyl orange or phenolphthalein.
- Add the other solution from the burette, swirling the conical flask until the indicator just changes colour. The volume should be recorded, reading to the bottom of the meniscus at eye level. This is a **rough titration**.
- Repeat the titration but add the solution **dropwise** near the end point and record the volume added. This is an accurate titration.
- Repeat the titration until the results are concordant (within 0.1 cm³ of each other).
- Calculate the mean of the accurate titrations.

The main steps to ensure **accuracy** in a titration include:

- rinsing the apparatus with the appropriate solution.
- adding the solution from the burette dropwise just before the end point.
- swirling the flask to make sure the reactants mix thoroughly and fully react.
- reading the burette at the bottom of the meniscus at eye level.
- to obtain **reliable** results the titration must be repeated and the mean of the accurate titrations, which should be concordant, calculated.

Titration results

To calculate the **mean titre**, do not use the rough titration. Use only concordant accurate titration values, and ignore any anomalies.

The table below shows a sample set of titration results. The titre is the **volume of solution** added from the burette. To work out the titre, subtract the initial burette reading from the final burette reading.

	Initial burette reading/ cm^3	Final burette reading/ cm^3	Titre/cm^3
Rough titration	0.0	24.5	24.5
Accurate titration 1	24.5	47.9	23.4
Accurate titration 2	0.0	23.3	23.3
Mean titre =	$\frac{23.4 + 23.3}{2}$		23.4

Note that the results are given to one decimal place in the table, so the mean titre must be given to one decimal place.

Titration calculations

The results of a titration can be used to calculate the concentration of a solution.

The steps to use in your calculation are:

- Underneath the balanced symbol equation, write the **information** (volume, concentration) given in the question and circle the substance that you need to find the concentration of.
- Calculate the number of **moles** of the solution added from the burette using:

$$\text{moles} = \frac{\text{volume (cm}^3) \times \text{conc (mol dm}^{-3})}{1000}$$

- Calculate the number of moles of the substance you need to find the concentration of using the **ratio** from the balanced symbol equation.
- Calculate the **concentration** using:

$$\frac{\text{concentration}}{\text{(mol dm}^{-3})} = \frac{\text{moles} \times 1000}{\text{volume (cm}^3)} \text{ of the substance.}$$

> **Tip:** You may be asked to give your answer to a given number of significant figures. The first significant figure of a number is the first digit that is not zero. For example, 0.046 has two significant figures, 60.0 has three significant figures, 21.34 has four significant figures. When rounding to a certain number of significant figures, if the next number is 5 or more round up, if the next number is 4 or less do not round up.

Worked example

In a titration, 25.0 cm^3 of sodium hydroxide solution reacted with 22.5 cm^3 of 0.500 mol dm^{-3} solution of sulfuric acid. Calculate the concentration of the sodium hydroxide solution in mol dm^{-3}.

Answer

$$H_2SO_4 + \boxed{2NaOH} \rightarrow Na_2SO_4 + 2H_2O$$

info: 22.5 cm^3 25.0 cm^3
0.500 mol dm^{-3}

$$\textbf{moles of } H_2SO_4 = \frac{\text{volume (cm}^3) \times \text{conc (mol dm}^{-3})}{1000} = \frac{22.5 \times 0.500}{1000} = 0.01125$$

ratio: 1 H_2SO_4 : 2NaOH
0.01125 : ?

There is twice the number of moles of NaOH as there is of H_2SO_4.

0.01125 : 2 × 0.01125
0.01125 : 0.0225

Hence there are 0.0225 moles of NaOH.

$$\textbf{concentration of NaOH in mol dm}^{-3} = \frac{\text{moles} \times 1000}{\text{vol (cm}^3)} = \frac{0.0225 \times 1000}{25.0} = 0.900 \text{ mol dm}^{-3}$$

Often questions are more structured than the example above, and are similar to the following worked examples.

3.2 VOLUMETRIC ANALYSIS

Worked example

25.0 cm³ of sodium hydroxide solution was pipetted into a conical flask and titrated with 0.400 mol dm⁻³ of sulfuric acid. 20.0 cm³ was needed to completely neutralise the sodium hydroxide solution. The equation for the reaction is:

$2NaOH + H_2SO_4 \rightarrow Na_2SO_4 + 2H_2O$

(a) Calculate the number of moles of sulfuric acid solution used in the titration.
(b) Calculate the number of moles of sodium hydroxide solution that reacted with the H_2SO_4.
(c) Calculate the concentration of the sodium hydroxide solution in mol dm⁻³.

Answer

info: (2NaOH)   + H_2SO_4 → Na_2SO_4 + $2H_2O$
        25.0 cm³   20.0 cm³
                      0.400 mol dm⁻³

(a) **moles** of H_2SO_4 = $\dfrac{\text{volume (cm}^3\text{)} \times \text{conc (mol dm}^{-3}\text{)}}{1000}$

$= \dfrac{20.0 \times 0.400}{1000}$

$= 0.008$ mol

(b) **ratio:** $1H_2SO_4 : 2NaOH$
    $0.008 : ?$

The ratio shows that there are twice as many moles of NaOH as H_2SO_4, so multiply the number of moles of H_2SO_4 by two.

$0.008 : 2 \times 0.008$
$= 0.016$ mol

(c) **concentration** of NaOH in mol dm⁻³ = $\dfrac{\text{moles} \times 1000}{\text{volume (cm}^3\text{)}}$

$= \dfrac{0.016 \times 1000}{25.0}$

$= 0.640$ mol dm⁻³

Worked example

25.0 cm³ of sulfuric acid solution was pipetted into a flask and titrated with 0.100 mol dm⁻³ potassium hydroxide solution. 22.5 cm³ of potassium hydroxide solution was needed to completely neutralise the acid.

$2KOH + H_2SO_4 \rightarrow K_2SO_4 + 2H_2O$

(a) Calculate the number of moles of potassium hydroxide solution used in the titration.
(b) Use your answer to (a) and the equation to calculate the concentration of the sulfuric acid.

Answer

$2KOH + H_2SO_4 \rightarrow K_2SO_4 + 2H_2O$

info: 22.5 cm³   25.0 cm³
0.100 mol dm⁻³

(a) **moles** of KOH $= \dfrac{\text{volume (cm}^3\text{)} \times \text{conc (mol dm}^{-3}\text{)}}{1000}$

$= \dfrac{22.5 \times 0.100}{1000}$

$= 0.00225$ mol

(b) **ratio:** 2 KOH : 1 H_2SO_4
0.00225 : ?

The number of moles of sulfuric acid is half the number of moles of KOH, so divide the number of moles of KOH by two.

0.00225 : 0.00225 ÷ 2
= 0.001125 mol

concentration in mol dm⁻³ $= \dfrac{\text{moles} \times 1000}{\text{volume (cm}^3\text{)}}$

$= \dfrac{0.001125 \times 1000}{25.0}$

$= 0.045$ mol dm⁻³

Questions

1. Calculate the concentration of the following solutions in mol dm⁻³:
   (a) 120 g of NaOH dissolved in 2 dm³ of solution. [2]
   (b) 3.4 g of NH_3 dissolved in 200 cm³ of solution. [2]
   (c) 5.3g of Na_2CO_3 dissolved in 250 cm³ of solution. [2]   **[6 marks]**

2. Calculate the number of moles of solute in:
   (a) 4 dm³ of 0.30 mol dm⁻³ HCl. [1]
   (b) 1.5 dm³ of 2.0 mol dm⁻³ HCl. [1]
   (c) 100 cm³ of 1.50 mol dm⁻³ NaOH. [1]
   (d) 25 cm³ of 0.50 mol dm⁻³ NaOH. [1]
   [4 marks]

3. 25.0 cm³ of sulfuric acid solution was placed in a conical flask and titrated with a standard solution of sodium hydroxide until the end point was reached.
   (a) What is a standard solution? [1]
   (b) Explain which indicator could be used in this titration and state the colour change at the end point. [4]   **[5 marks]**

4. To prepare a standard solution of sodium hydroxide, a student weighed out 1.8 g of sodium hydroxide and used a 250 cm³ volumetric flask to make up the solution.
   (a) What is the concentration, in mol dm⁻³, of the standard solution of sodium hydroxide that the student prepared? [2]
   (b) Describe the method the student used to prepare the standard solution of sodium hydroxide. [6] **[8 marks]**

5. In a titration, 20.0 cm³ of a solution of sulfuric acid reacted with 16.4 cm³ of 0.400 mol dm⁻³ sodium hydroxide solution.
   (a) Find the concentration of the sulfuric acid in mol dm⁻³. The equation for the reaction is:
   $$H_2SO_4 + 2NaOH \rightarrow Na_2SO_4 + 2H_2O \quad [3]$$
   (b) Explain why phenolphthalein is a suitable indicator to use in this titration. [1] **[4 marks]**

6. 25.0 cm³ of calcium hydroxide solution was placed in a conical flask and completely reacted with 19.8 cm³ of 0.0500 mol dm⁻³ hydrochloric acid solution in a titration. The equation for the reaction is:
   $$2HCl + Ca(OH)_2 \rightarrow CaCl_2 + 2H_2O$$
   (a) Calculate the number of moles of hydrochloric acid used in the titration. [1]
   (b) Calculate the number of moles of calcium hydroxide present in 25.0 cm³ of the solution in the conical flask. [1]
   (c) Calculate the number of moles of calcium hydroxide present in 1000.0 cm³ of the solution. [1] **[3 marks]**

7. 25.0 cm³ of barium hydroxide solution was titrated with a solution of hydrochloric acid of concentration 0.200 mol dm⁻³. The balanced symbol equation for the reaction is:
   $$Ba(OH)_2 + 2HCl \rightarrow BaCl_2 + 2H_2O$$
   (a) Describe how you would accurately measure out and transfer 25.0 cm³ of barium hydroxide solution into a conical flask. [4]
   (b) Describe in detail how you would prepare and fill the burette and carry out a titration using a named indicator to determine the volume of hydrochloric acid required to neutralise the 25.0 cm³ of barium hydroxide. [8]
   (c) The results from the titration are shown in the table below.

	Initial burette reading/ cm³	Final burette reading/ cm³	Titre/ cm³
Rough	0.0	23.1	23.1
1st accurate	23.2	45.5	
2nd accurate	0.0	22.4	

   (i) Complete the results table above. [1]
   (ii) Calculate the mean titre from the results. [1]
   (iii) Calculate the number of moles of hydrochloric acid used in this titration. [1]
   (iv) Use the balanced symbol equation to work out the number of moles of barium hydroxide that reacted with the hydrochloric acid. [1]
   (v) Calculate the concentration of barium hydroxide in mol dm⁻³. [1] **[17 marks]**

8. In a titration, 25.0 cm³ of sodium carbonate solution was titrated with 0.100 mol dm⁻³ of hydrochloric acid and the mean titre was 12.4 cm³.
   (a) Calculate the moles of hydrochloric acid used in the titration. [1]
   (b) Calculate the moles of sodium carbonate that completely reacted with the acid using the chemical equation below:
   $$2HCl + Na_2CO_3 \rightarrow 2NaCl + H_2O + CO_2 \quad [1]$$
   (c) Calculate the concentration of the sodium carbonate solution in mol dm⁻³. [1] **[3 marks]**

3.3 ENERGETICS

Students should be able to:

3.3.1 demonstrate an understanding of the reasons why chemical reactions usually involve heat change;

3.3.2 contrast the terms exothermic and endothermic;

3.3.3 define the term standard enthalpy change ($\Delta H^\ominus$), standard enthalpy of combustion ($\Delta_c H^\ominus$), standard enthalpy of formation ($\Delta_f H^\ominus$) and standard enthalpy of neutralisation ($\Delta_n H^\ominus$);

3.3.4 recall standard conditions as 100 kPa and 298 K;

3.3.5 demonstrate knowledge of enthalpy changes in combustion and neutralisation reactions;

3.3.6 describe common experimental methods to determine the enthalpy change in a combustion and a neutralisation reaction;

3.3.7 recall and use the equation $Q = mc\Delta T$ to calculate enthalpy changes in a reaction;

3.3.8 explain the concept of the principle of conservation of energy;

3.3.9 define Hess's law;

3.3.10 construct simple enthalpy cycles and use these to carry out simple enthalpy change calculations;

3.3.11 explain the term average bond enthalpy;

3.3.12 use average bond enthalpies to calculate the enthalpy change of a reaction; and

3.3.13 account for the differences between theoretical and experimental bond enthalpy values.

Exothermic and endothermic reactions

An **exothermic reaction** is one in which **heat energy is given out**. This means that the surroundings become hotter and the temperature rises. An exothermic reaction has a **negative** energy change value.

> **Tip: Ex**othermic heat is given out – heat '**ex**its.'

Neutralisation reactions and combustion reactions are exothermic. Fuels burning, such as methane (CH_4) in natural gas, are very exothermic combustion reactions. They release a lot of heat energy and catch fire.

An **endothermic reaction** is one in which **heat energy is taken in**. The temperature of the surroundings drops. An endothermic reaction has a **positive** energy change value. Endothermic reactions are less common than exothermic reactions. Thermal decomposition reactions are endothermic.

Enthalpy change

Enthalpy (H) is the heat content that is stored in a chemical reaction. Enthalpy of reactants and products cannot be measured directly but the energy absorbed or released during a reaction can be measured – this is the **enthalpy change** (ΔH) (delta H). Enthalpy change varies depending on the conditions, so standard enthalpy changes ($\Delta H^\ominus$) are measured under standard conditions.

> **Tip:** The $\ominus$ symbol means standard.

Standard enthalpy change ($\Delta H^\ominus$) is the change in heat energy in a reaction, at constant pressure.

Standard conditions are:
- **298 K (25°C)**
- **a pressure of 100 kPa**

Note that temperature can be given in degrees Celsius (°C) or in kelvin. Temperature in kelvin = temperature in degrees Celsius + 273.

You will learn about standard enthalpy of combustion, neutralisation and formation in this chapter.

Why do chemical reactions involve a change in heat energy?

Breaking a chemical bond takes in energy. Making a chemical bond releases energy. Bond **breaking** is endothermic and has a **positive** enthalpy value. Bond **making** is exothermic and has a **negative** enthalpy value.

For example, 348 kJ (kilojoules) of energy is taken in to break one mole of C–C covalent bonds and this is written as +348 kJ mol^{-1}. Making one mole of C–C covalent bonds releases 348 kJ of energy and this is written as –348 kJ mol^{-1}.

3.3 ENERGETICS

During a chemical reaction:
- energy must be taken in to break bonds in the reactants.
- energy is given out when bonds in the products are formed.

The overall energy change for a reaction equals the difference between the energy taken in to break the bonds in the reactants and the energy released when bonds are formed in the products.

energy change = energy taken in breaking bonds in reactants − energy released making bonds in products

	Exothermic reaction	Endothermic reaction
Comparison of bond energies	More energy is released making new bonds than is taken in to break bonds	More energy is taken in to break bonds than is released making new bonds
Sign of energy change	−	+

To explain why a reaction is exothermic or endothermic:
- state that bond breaking takes in energy and name the reactants in which the bonds are broken.
- state that bond making gives out energy and name the reactants in which the bonds are made.
- compare the two energies and state which is greater.

Worked example
Propane burns in oxygen, releasing energy:

propane + oxygen → carbon dioxide + water

Explain why the reaction is exothermic, in terms of the energy of the bonds.

Answer
- The energy taken in to break the bonds in propane and oxygen
- is less than
- the energy given out when bonds are made in carbon dioxide and water.

Worked example
The reaction of hydrogen with iodine to form hydrogen iodide is endothermic:

$H_2 + I_2 \rightarrow 2HI$

Explain why this reaction is endothermic in terms of the energy of the bonds.

Answer
- The energy taken in to break bonds in H_2 and I_2
- is greater than
- the energy given out when bonds are made in HI.

Reaction profiles

Chemical reactions can only occur when particles collide with each other with enough energy to react. **The activation energy (E_a) is the minimum energy needed for a reaction to occur.**

A reaction profile is a graph that shows the relative energy of the reactants and products in a reaction. It can also show the activation energy (E_a). The reaction pathway is shown as a line from reactants to products. Reaction pathways require an input of energy to break bonds in the reactants before new bonds can form in the products. This is the minimum amount of energy needed for a reaction to occur (activation energy E_a).

Tip: Make sure you can draw and label a reaction profile diagram for an exothermic and an endothermic reaction. This is mentioned in section 3.4.2 of the specification.

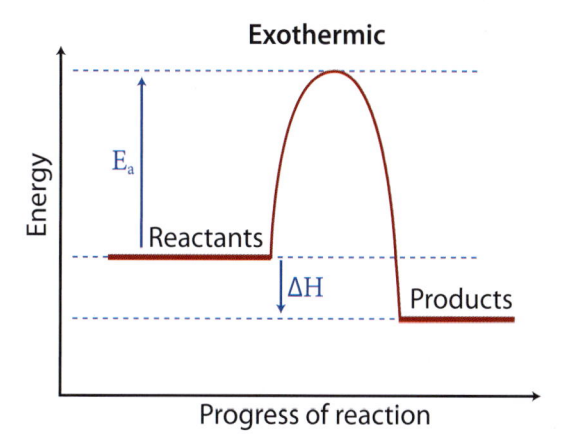

Exothermic reaction profile

Endothermic reaction profile

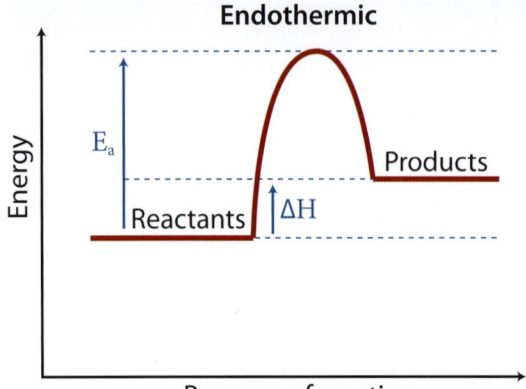

Note that for an exothermic reaction, the products have less energy than reactants, as heat has been given out. This means the overall enthalpy change (ΔH) is negative. For an endothermic reaction, the products have more energy than the reactants, and are at a higher level on the reaction profile, as heat energy has been taken in. This means the overall enthalpy change (ΔH) is positive.

Average bond enthalpy

Average bond enthalpies relate to the strength of a covalent bond. A higher bond enthalpy value means a stronger covalent bond.

Average bond enthalpy is the energy required to break one mole of a given bond averaged over many compounds.

The unit of average bond enthalpy is kJ mol^{-1}.

To calculate the enthalpy change in a reaction, the method is as follows:

- Calculate the total average bond enthalpies for all the bonds broken in the reactants.
- Calculate the total average bond enthalpies for all the bonds made in the reactants.
- Use the equation shown below.

enthalpy change = energy taken in breaking bonds in reactants − energy released making bonds in products

Worked example
Draw a labelled reaction profile diagram for the reaction shown:

$CH_4 + 2O_2 \rightarrow CO_2 + 2H_2O$

The enthalpy change for the reaction is −890 kJ mol^{-1}.

Answer
The enthalpy change is negative so it is an exothermic reaction.
Draw the general shape of an exothermic reaction profile.
Then label the reactants (CH_4 and $2O_2$) and the products (CO_2 and $2H_2O$).

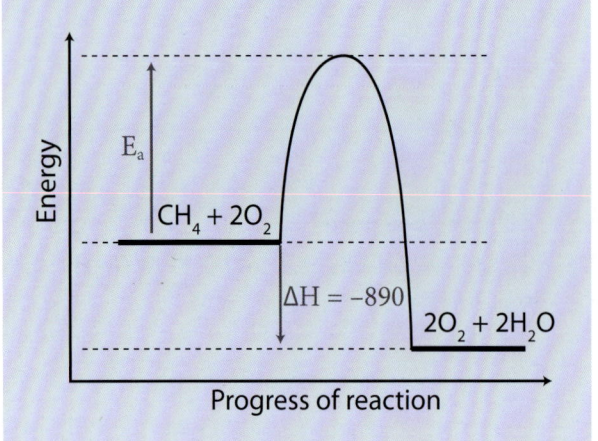

Worked example
Calculate the enthalpy change in the following reaction using the average bond energies given.

average bond enthalpy in kJ mol^{-1}:

C–H = 412, O=O = 496, C=O = 743, O–H = 463

H–C(H)(H)–H + 2 O=O → O=C=O + 2 O(H)(H)

Answer

bonds broken = 4C–H + 2O=O
= (4 × 412) + (2 × 496)
= 2640

bonds made = 2C=O + 4O–H
= (2 × 743) + (4 × 463)
= 3338

enthalpy change (ΔH) = energy taken in breaking bonds − energy released making bonds

ΔH = 2640 − 3338
= −698 kJ mol^{-1}

3.3 ENERGETICS

Worked example
Calculate the enthalpy change for the following reaction using the average bond enthalpies given:

average bond enthalpy in kJ mol^{-1}: C–H = 412, O=O = 496, C=O = 743, O–H = 463, C–C = 348

$$CH_3-CH_2-CH_3 + 5\,O=O \rightarrow 3\,O=C=O + 4\,H-O-H$$

Answer
bonds broken = 8C–H + 2C–C + 5O=O
= (8 × 412) + (2 × 348) + (5 × 496)
= 3296 + 696 + 2480
= 6472

bonds made = 6C=O + 8O–H
= (6 × 743) + (8 × 463)
= 4458 + 3704
= 8162

ΔH = 6472 – 8162 = –1690 kJ mol^{-1}

*This reaction has a **more** exothermic enthalpy change than the reaction in the previous example as **more bonds** are broken and made.*

Worked example
Hydrogen reacts with oxygen in an exothermic reaction.

H–H + ½ O=O → H–O–H

ΔH = –242 kJ mol^{-1}

Calculate the average bond enthalpy of the H–H bond.

average bond enthalpy in kJ mol^{-1}: O=O = 496, O–H = 463

Answer
bonds broken = H–H + ½O=O
= H–H + ½ × 496
= H–H + 248

bonds made = 2O–H
= 2 × 463
= 926

enthalpy change (ΔH) = energy taken in breaking bonds – energy released making bonds

This time the ΔH value is given in the question.

–242 = H–H + 248 – 926
H–H = 926 – 248 – 242 = +436 kJ mol^{-1}

Enthalpy changes determined from average bond enthalpies (theoretical bond energies) **often differ** from **experimentally** determined values. This is because the average bond enthalpies are not specific to the bonds in the molecules involved but are **averaged across many different molecules** containing that particular bond. For example, the average bond enthalpy value of C–Cl bond is 339 kJ mol^{-1}, however, in the CCl_4 molecule, the actual C–Cl bond enthalpy value is 329 and in the CH_3Cl molecule, the value is 334 kJ mol^{-1}. Also, for standard enthalpy changes, water would be a liquid, but when using mean bond enthalpies, the substances are in the gaseous state.

Experimental method to determine the enthalpy change of combustion

Combustion is a reaction in which a substance reacts with oxygen to form oxides and release energy.

Enthalpy change of combustion ($\Delta_c H^\circ$), is the enthalpy change when 1 mole of a substance is completely burnt in oxygen (under standard conditions).

For example, an equation for the standard enthalpy change of combustion for methane (CH_4) is:

$$CH_{4(g)} + 2O_{2(g)} \rightarrow CO_{2(g)} + 2H_2O_{(l)}$$

or for ethanol (C_2H_5OH):

$$C_2H_5OH_{(l)} + 3O_{2(g)} \rightarrow 2CO_{2(g)} + 3H_2O_{(l)}$$

or for hydrogen:

$$H_{2(g)} + ½O_{2(g)} \rightarrow H_2O_{(l)}$$

Note that this is balanced with ½ mole of oxygen as **one mole** of the substance (hydrogen) burns in enthalpy of combustion.

The simple apparatus used to measure the enthalpy change of combustion of a liquid fuel is shown in the diagram below. The method is:

- Burn a known mass of substance in air and use it to heat a known mass of water.
- Measure the temperature change in the water.

To calculate the enthalpy change, the equation:

$$Q = mc\Delta T$$

is used where
Q = heat energy change in J (joules)
m = mass of water heated in g
c = specific heat capacity of water (4.2 J g^{-1} K^{-1})
ΔT = temperature change in kelvin (K) or °C

> **Tip:** Specific heat capacity is the heat required to raise the temperature of 1 g of a given substance by one degree.

The calorimeter is usually a copper can. The method to determine the enthalpy of combustion of a liquid fuel such as ethanol or methanol is:

- Measure a volume of water (e.g. 100 cm³) into a calorimeter/beaker using a measuring cylinder. (100 cm³ is the same as 100 g of water as the density of water is 1 g/cm³).
- Weigh a spirit burner containing the liquid fuel to be burnt.
- Measure the initial temperature of water using a thermometer (T_1).
- Place the spirit burner under the calorimeter and light the wick.
- Use the spirit burner to heat the water.
- When there is a reasonable temperature rise (15°C), stop heating and extinguish the flame. Stir and measure the final temperature (T_2) of the water using a thermometer.
- Cool and reweigh the spirit burner.
- Calculate temperature change (ΔT) = $T_2 - T_1$ and the heat energy change in joules using $Q = mc\Delta T$.
- Calculate the mass of fuel used in the burner by subtraction, and calculate the number of moles of fuel used using:

$$\text{moles} = \frac{\text{mass (g)}}{M_r}$$

- Calculate the energy change per mole of fuel used:

$$\left(\frac{Q}{\text{number of moles of fuel burnt}}\right)$$

> **Tip:** Note that the enthalpy change of combustion is negative, and the temperature of the water rises, so the **highest** temperature reached is recorded.

> **Tip:** It is a good idea to repeat the experiment using a fresh 100 cm³ of water and average the results.

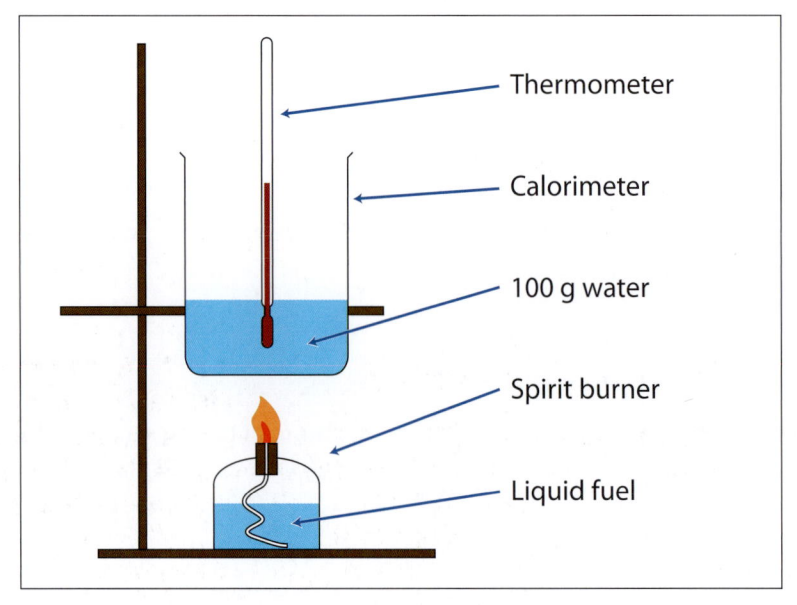

Experimental determination of enthalpy of combustion of a liquid fuel

3.3 ENERGETICS

Worked example
In an experiment to determine the enthalpy change of combustion of butan-1-ol (C_4H_9OH) the following results were obtained.

mass of burner + butan-1-ol = 55.40 g
mass of burner + butan-1-ol after burning = 53.89 g
initial temperature of water = 20.2°C
final temperature of water = 44.4°C
mass of water in calorimeter = 100 g

Calculate the enthalpy change of combustion of butan-1-ol. The specific heat capacity of water is 4.2 J g^{-1} °C^{-1}.

Answer
First find the number of moles of fuel burned:

mass of butan-1-ol burned = 55.40 − 53.89
= 1.51 g

M_r butan-1-ol = (4 × relative atomic mass of carbon) + (10 × relative atomic mass of hydrogen) + (1 × relative atomic mass of oxygen)

= (4 × 12) + (10 × 1) + (1 × 16)
= 74

moles of butan-1-ol = $\dfrac{\text{mass (g)}}{M_r}$ = $\dfrac{1.51}{74}$
= 0.02041 mol

Next, find the energy change during the experiment:

temperature change = 44.4 − 20.2 = 24.2°C
$Q = mc\Delta T = 100 \times 4.2 \times 24.2 = -10164$ J

Note that this an exothermic reaction and heat is given out, so a negative sign must be included.

Then work out the enthalpy change per mole in J mol^{-1} by dividing the value of Q by the number of moles and convert to kJ mol^{-1} by dividing by 1000.

enthalpy change of combustion = $\dfrac{-10164}{0.02041}$

= −497991.18 J mol^{-1}
= −498 kJ mol^{-1}

> **Tip:** Remember to include the sign for the enthalpy change. Here it is a − sign as it is an **exothermic** reaction.

When carrying out this experiment it is assumed that all the energy is transferred to the water and no heat energy is lost. However this is not the case. The value for the enthalpy change of combustion determined experimentally is frequently **less exothermic** than the value found in data books. This is because of sources of error in the experiment due to:

- heat loss to the surroundings from the spirit burner, wick and calorimeter (e.g. the flame is affected by draughts).
- heat gain by the calorimeter/copper can.
- incomplete combustion of the fuel, leaving soot on the bottom of the calorimeter.
- fuel loss from the wick or burner by evaporation.
- water loss by evaporation.
- the reaction being unlikely to occur under standard conditions, especially temperature.

Simple experiments can be **improved** to obtain more accurate values by:

- using a draught shield to reduce heat loss to the surroundings.
- using a lid on the calorimeter to reduce heat loss to the surroundings.
- minimising the distance between the flame and the calorimeter.
- insulating the calorimeter and the spirit burner to reduce heat loss.
- using a top on the spirit burner with wick protruding to minimise evaporation.
- if possible, burning in a supply of pure oxygen to prevent incomplete combustion.

Experimental determination of enthalpy change of neutralisation

Enthalpy change of neutralisation ($\Delta_n H^\ominus$) is the enthalpy change when one mole of water is produced in a neutralisation (under standard conditions). For example, an equation for the standard enthalpy change of neutralisation for the reaction of sodium hydroxide and hydrochloric acid is:

$NaOH_{(aq)} + HCl_{(aq)} \rightarrow NaCl_{(aq)} + H_2O_{(l)}$

The equation for the standard enthalpy change of neutralisation for the reaction of sodium hydroxide and sulfuric acid is:

$NaOH_{(aq)} + ½H_2SO_{4(aq)} \rightarrow ½Na_2SO_{4(aq)} + H_2O_{(l)}$

Note that the equation must be balanced using ½ mole of sulfuric acid, as, by definition, standard enthalpy of neutralisation is for one mole of water being produced.

Enthalpy changes in solution, such as enthalpy change of neutralisation, can be measured using insulated plastic cups as calorimeters, as shown in the diagram below. The temperature of the acid before mixing is recorded, followed by the maximum temperature of the solution after adding the alkali. The temperature difference is calculated.

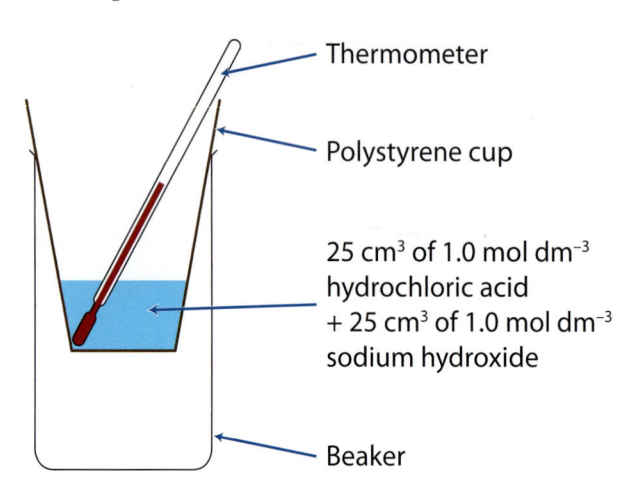

Determining enthalpy of neutralisation

The **method** to determine the enthalpy change of neutralisation is:

- Place a polystyrene cup in a glass beaker for support (the beaker also provides extra insulation and prevents draughts).
- Rinse a measuring cylinder with 1.0 mol dm⁻³ HCl and then measure 25 cm³ of HCl and transfer into the polystyrene cup.

Tip: If you are measuring out 25.0 cm³ rather than 25 cm³ you need to use a more accurate measuring device such as a pipette or burette.

- Stir the acid with a thermometer and record the temperature (T_1).
- Rinse a second measuring cylinder with 1.0 mol dm⁻³ $NaOH_{(aq)}$ and then measure out 25 cm³ of $NaOH_{(aq)}$.
- Add the $NaOH_{(aq)}$ to the acid, stir and record the highest temperature reached (T_2).

- Calculate temperature change (ΔT) = $T_2 - T_1$ and the heat energy change in joules using $Q = mc\Delta T$
- Calculate the number of moles of acid used, the number of moles of water formed and the enthalpy of neutralisation.

Tip: Note that the enthalpy of neutralisation for acid and alkali is negative, as the temperature increases and it is the **highest** temperature reached that is recorded.

Worked example

25 cm³ of 2.00 mol dm⁻³ hydrochloric acid was mixed with 25 cm³ of 2.00 mol dm⁻³ sodium hydroxide solution in a polystyrene cup. The temperature changed from 22.5°C to 34.5°C. Calculate the enthalpy change of this neutralisation reaction.

$HCl_{(aq)} + NaOH_{(aq)} \rightarrow NaCl_{(aq)} + H_2O_{(aq)}$

Answer

Enthalpy change of neutralisation is the enthalpy change when one mole of water is produced in a neutralisation.

First find the number of moles of water produced.

$$\text{moles of HCl} = \frac{\text{vol (cm}^3\text{)} \times \text{conc}}{1000}$$

$$= \frac{25 \times 2.00}{1000}$$

$$= 0.050$$

$$\text{moles of NaOH} = \frac{\text{vol (cm}^3\text{)} \times \text{conc}}{1000}$$

$$= \frac{25 \times 2.00}{1000}$$

$$= 0.050$$

There are the same moles of acid and alkali in the cup, and so both are completely used up in reaction. Due to the 1:1 ratio in the balanced symbol equation:

moles acid = moles alkali = moles water

moles of water = 0.050

Next, find the energy change during the experiment:

temperature change = 34.5 − 22.5 = 12.0°C

mass of solution in the cup = 25 + 25 = 50 g

3.3 ENERGETICS

$Q = mc\Delta T = 50 \times 4.2 \times 12.0 = -2520$ J

Note that this an exothermic reaction so a negative sign must be included.

Then work out the enthalpy change per mole in J mol^{-1} by dividing the value of Q by the number of moles, and then in kJ mol^{-1} by dividing by 1000.

$$\text{enthalpy change of neutralisation} = \frac{-2520}{0.050}$$
$$= -50400 \text{ J mol}^{-1}$$
$$= -50.4 \text{ kJ mol}^{-1}$$

Tip: Remember to include the sign for the enthalpy change. Here it is a – sign as it is an **exothermic** reaction.

Sometimes a reaction may be **endothermic**, so heat is taken in. The temperature falls, and thus in the experimental method, the **lowest temperature** reached must be recorded. The next example is for an endothermic reaction.

Worked example
To determine the enthalpy of change of the reaction between potassium hydrogencarbonate and sulfuric acid, a student added 5.0 g of potassium hydrogencarbonate to 50.0 cm^3 of 2.0 mol dm^{-3} sulfuric acid in a polystyrene cup.

(a) Name three pieces of apparatus that are used to take measurements in this experiment.

Answer
- Balance (to weigh the potassium hydrogencarbonate)
- Pipette/burette (to measure 50.0 cm^3 of sulfuric acid)
- Thermometer (to measure the temperature change)

(b) Describe the method used. Include the pieces of apparatus named in (a) and the measurements taken.

Answer
- Weigh 5.0 g of potassium hydrogencarbonate using a balance.
- Transfer 50.0 cm^3 of sulfuric acid (an excess) into a polystyrene cup using a burette/pipette.
- Measure the initial temperature of the acid using a thermometer.
- Add the potassium hydrogencarbonate to the acid.
- Stir with the thermometer.
- Measure the lowest temperature reached.

Tip: For an **endothermic** reaction, the polystyrene cup is used to minimise **heat gain** from surroundings. For an **exothermic** reaction, the polystyrene cup is used to minimise **heat loss** to the surroundings.

Worked example
A student added 5.0 g of potassium hydrogencarbonate (KHCO$_3$) to 50.0 cm^3 of 2.0 mol dm^{-3} sulfuric acid (an excess) and the temperature fell from 18°C to 10°C.

Use the equation $Q = m \times 4.2 \times \Delta T$, to calculate the value of Q and then the enthalpy change for the reaction.

Answer
First find the number of moles of potassium hydrogen carbonate used.

M_r KHCO$_3$ = 39 + 1 + 12 + (3 × 16) = 100

$$\text{moles} = \frac{\text{mass (g)}}{M_r} = \frac{5.0}{100} = 0.050 \text{ mol}$$

Next, find the energy change during the experiment.

temperature change = 18 – 10 = 8°C
$Q = m \times 4.2 \times \Delta T = 50.0 \times 4.2 \times 8$
= +1680 J

Note that this is an endothermic reaction, so heat has been taken in and the temperature has dropped, so a plus sign must be included.

Then work out the enthalpy change per mole in J mol^{-1} by dividing the value of Q by the number of moles and then in kJ mol^{-1} by dividing by 1000.

$$\text{enthalpy change} = \frac{1680}{0.050} = +33600 \text{ J mol}^{-1}$$
$$= +33.6 \text{ kJ mol}^{-1}$$

Tip: Remember to include the sign for the enthalpy change. This time it is a + sign as it is an **endothermic** reaction.

Simple enthalpy cycles to calculate the enthalpy change of a reaction

Hess's law states that the enthalpy change for a reaction is independent of the route taken, provided the initial and final conditions are the same.

Hess's law is an application of the **principle of the conservation of energy**, which states that **energy cannot be created or destroyed but it can change from one form to another**.

It is often difficult to find enthalpy changes experimentally, so they can be found indirectly, by calculation using Hess's law and known values of enthalpy of combustion or enthalpy of formation.

Standard enthalpy change of formation ($\Delta_f H^\ominus$) is the enthalpy change when one mole of a compound is formed from its elements under standard conditions.

For example, for water the equation for enthalpy of formation (forming one mole) is:

$$H_{2(g)} + \tfrac{1}{2}O_{2(g)} \rightarrow H_2O_{(l)}$$

or for ethanol:

$$2C_{(s)} + \tfrac{1}{2}O_{2(g)} + 3H_{2(g)} \rightarrow C_2H_5OH_{(l)}$$

Standard enthalpy of combustion ($\Delta_c H$) and standard enthalpy of formation ($\Delta_f H$) values can both be used in cycles to calculate enthalpy changes. The cycle is different depending on the data used.

1. Calculation of an enthalpy change using standard enthalpy of combustion values

The cycle shown below can be used to calculate the enthalpy of a reaction, using Hess's law.

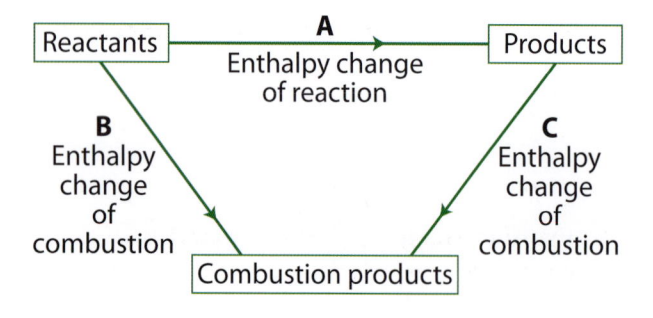

```
          A
Reactants ───→ Products
          Enthalpy change
          of reaction
    B              C
Enthalpy         Enthalpy
change           change
of               of
combustion       combustion
       ↘       ↙
    Combustion products
```

There are two different routes to get from reactants to products:

Route 1 = A

Route 2 = B − C

By Hess's law the total enthalpy change is the same for each route so:

A = B − C

Worked example

Calculate the enthalpy change for the reaction:

$$3C_{(s)} + 4H_{2(g)} \rightarrow C_3H_{8(g)}$$

using the enthalpy of combustion data shown in the table below:

Substance	Enthalpy of combustion (kJ mol^{-1})
$C_{(s)}$	−394
$H_{2(g)}$	−286
$C_3H_{8(g)}$	−2219

Answer

First draw the cycle, inserting all the enthalpy of combustion values. Remember to multiply by the balancing number in the equation.

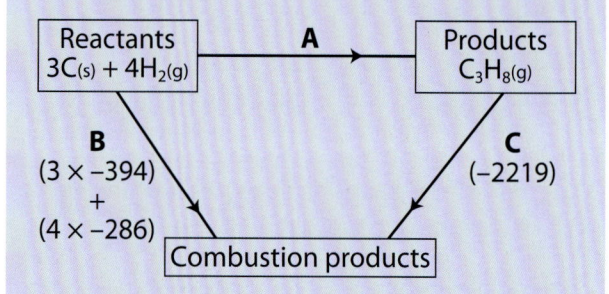

```
Reactants          A         Products
3C(s) + 4H2(g) ───────→      C3H8(g)
    B                           C
 (3 × −394)                  (−2219)
   +
 (4 × −286)
       ↘                    ↙
        Combustion products
```

Then use Hess's law:

Route 1 = A

Route 2 = B − C

A = B − C

A = [(3 × −394) + (4 × −286)] − [(−2219)]

A = (−1182) + (−1144) + 2219

A = −107 kJ mol^{-1}

ΔH = −107 kJ mol^{-1}

Tip: For enthalpy cycles using combustion data, the direction of the arrows goes from reactants to combustion products, and from products to combustion products.

3.3 ENERGETICS

2. Calculation of an enthalpy change using standard enthalpy of formation data

The cycle shown can be used to calculate the enthalpy of a reaction, using Hess's law.

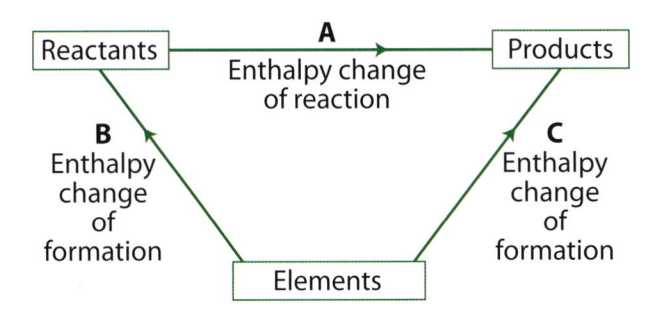

```
              A
Reactants ─────────────→ Products
         Enthalpy change
           of reaction
    B  ↖               ↗  C
   Enthalpy         Enthalpy
   change           change
   of               of
   formation        formation
            Elements
```

Note that the **direction** of arrows is **different** for this cycle, the enthalpy of formation is the enthalpy change to form a substance from its elements in their standard states, so the arrows go up.

There are two different routes to get from reactants to products:

Route 1 = A

Route 2 = –B + C = C – B

By Hess's law the total enthalpy change is the same for each route so:

A = –B + C

Worked example

Calculate the enthalpy change of reaction for:

$CH_{4(g)} + 2O_{2(g)} \rightarrow CO_{2(g)} + 2H_2O_{(g)}$

using the enthalpy of formation values given in the equation.

Substance	Enthalpy of formation / kJ mol⁻¹
CO_2	–394
H_2O	–286
CH_4	–76

Tip: O_2 is an element and has no enthalpy of formation value.

Answer

First draw the cycle, inserting all the enthalpy of combustion values. Remember to multiply by the balancing number in the equation.

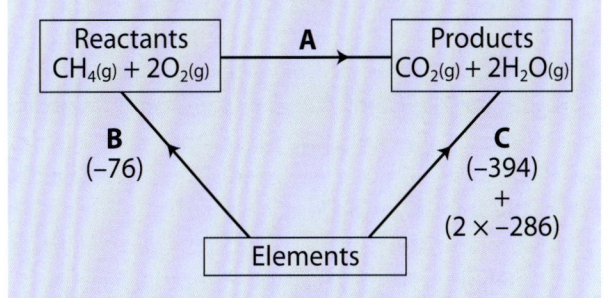

```
Reactants          A          Products
CH₄(g) + 2O₂(g) ─────→ CO₂(g) + 2H₂O(g)
       B  ↖              ↗  C
       (–76)           (–394)
                          +
                      (2 × –286)
              Elements
```

Then use Hess's law:

Route 1 = A

Route 2 = –B + C

A = –B + C

B = –(–76)

C = (–394) + (2 × –286)

A = –B + C

    = +76 – 394 – 572

    = –890 kJ mol⁻¹

ΔH = –890 kJ mol⁻¹

Tip: To succeed with these types of calculation you need to learn the two different cycles and remember the correct directions of arrows – **towards** combustion products, and **away** from elements.

Questions

1. State two differences between an exothermic reaction and endothermic reaction. **[2 marks]**

2. What are standard conditions? **[2 marks]**

3. Photosynthesis is shown by the word equation:

   carbon dioxide + water → glucose + oxygen

   Explain in terms of bonds why this is an endothermic reaction. **[3 marks]**

4. Define the term activation energy. **[1 mark]**

77

5. Draw a reaction profile for an exothermic reaction. Label the axes, the activation energy and the overall energy change. [4 marks]

6. (a) Define the term average bond enthalpy. [2]
   (b) The combustion of ethanol is represented by the equation:

   H H
   | |
   H—C—C—O—H + 3 O=O
   | |
   H H

   → 2 O=C=O + 3 H—O—H

   Calculate the value of the enthalpy change of combustion of ethanol using the bond enthalpy values: C–H = 412, C–C = 348, C–O = 264, O–H = 463, O=O = 496, C=O = 803 kJ mol^{-1} [3]
   (c) Why is the value calculated in (b) different from the experimentally determined value? [1]
   (d) Define enthalpy change of combustion. [2]
   (e) Describe the experimental method to determine the enthalpy change of combustion of ethanol, in the laboratory. [8]
   [16 marks]

7. The enthalpy change for the reaction
   $H_2 + Cl_2 \rightarrow 2HCl$ is -186 kJ mol^{-1}.
   Calculate a value for the bond enthalpy of the H–Cl bond using the following average bond enthalpies: H–H = 436, Cl–Cl = 242 kJ mol^{-1}. [4]
   [4 marks]

8. In an experiment 1.54 g of an alcohol with formula $C_5H_{12}O$ is burnt in a spirit burner underneath a beaker of water. The heat produced increases the temperature of 180 g of water from 22.8°C to 75.3°C.
   (a) Calculate the number of moles of the alcohol. [2]
   (b) Calculate the enthalpy change of combustion of the alcohol in kJ mol^{-1}. Give your answer to three significant figures. (Specific heat capacity of water = 4.18 J kg^{-1} °C) [4]
   (c) The value determined experimentally is different from the value given in data books. Suggest two reasons why the value is different. [2]
   (d) The complete combustion of the alcohol is represented by the equation:
   $C_5H_{12}O + 7 \frac{1}{2} O_2 \rightarrow 5CO_2 + 6H_2O$

   Enthalpy changes of formation are shown in the table below:

Substance	$C_5H_{12}O$	CO_2	H_2O
Enthalpy of formation/kJ mol^{-1}	−366	−394	−286

   Calculate the enthalpy change of combustion of the alcohol. [3]
   [11 marks]

9. Calculate the enthalpy change for the reaction:
   $C_2H_5OH + 3O_2 \rightarrow 2CO_2 + 3H_2O$
   Use the following enthalpy of formation values: Δ_fH° $C_2H_5OH = -277$, Δ_fH° $CO_2 = -394$, Δ_fH° $H_2O = -286$ kJ mol^{-1}
   [3 marks]

10. Calculate the enthalpy change for the reaction:
    $4C_{(s)} + 5H_{2(g)} \rightarrow C_4H_{10(g)}$
    Use the following enthalpy of combustion values: Δ_cH° $C_4H_{10} = -2880$, Δ_cH° C = −394, Δ_cH° $H_2 = -286$ kJ mol^{-1}
    [3 marks]

3.4 KINETICS

Students should be able to:

3.4.1 define the terms rate of reaction and activation energy;

3.4.2 construct a reaction profile diagram;

3.4.3 explain the factors that affect the rate of a reaction, including concentration, pressure of gases, temperature and use of a catalyst;

3.4.4 explain common practical techniques to follow the rate of a reaction and analyse the effects of these factors;

3.4.5 demonstrate an understanding of collision theory;

3.4.6 recall and use the Maxwell-Boltzmann distribution curve to explain the effects of change in temperature and action of a catalyst on the rate of a given reaction;

3.4.7 describe the process of chemisorption in catalysis;

3.4.8 define the term catalyst and describe the role of a catalyst in a catalytic converter, including the concept of catalyst poisoning;

3.4.9 demonstrate an understanding of the use of a solid (heterogeneous) catalyst for industrial reactions; and

3.4.10 evaluate the economic benefits of using catalysts in industrial reactions, including the manufacture of ammonia, sulfuric acid and nitric acid.

Rate of reaction

The rate of a reaction is a measure of the speed at which reactants are changed into products.

In a fast reaction it takes a **short** time to convert reactants to products. Dynamite exploding and potassium reacting with water are examples of fast reactions. In a slow reaction it takes a **long** time to convert reactants to products. Rusting of iron is a slow reaction.

rate of reaction =
$\dfrac{\text{quantity of reactant used or product formed}}{\text{time taken}}$

Tip: Reaction profiles for exothermic and endothermic reactions (as shown on pages 69–70) should also be revised for this topic.

Collision theory

Collision theory states that for a reaction to occur the reacting particles (these may be atoms, ions or molecules) must collide together with enough energy to react. **Activation energy (E_a) is the minimum energy needed for a reaction to occur.**

Successful collisions are ones that result in a reaction, and they take place when reactant particles collide with the activation energy. The activation energy is used to help break bonds so that the atoms can be rearranged to make products. Unsuccessful collisions are collisions that do not result in reaction and occur when the particles collide with less than the activation energy.

In general, reaction rates are increased when the frequency and energy of the collisions is increased.

Tip: Frequency is the number of collisions in a certain amount of time.

Factors affecting the rate of reactions

Various factors can change the rate of a reaction, including:

1. Concentration of solution

Increasing the concentration of a solution increases the rate of reaction.

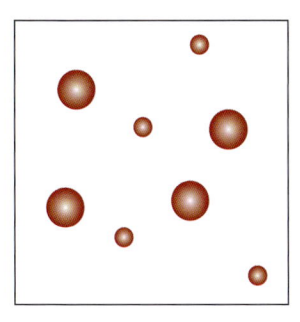

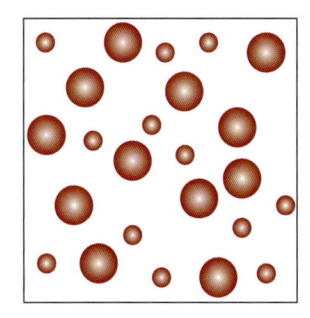

Low concentration   High concentration

Explanation:
- There are more particles present in the same volume.
- This results in more successful collisions (with the activation energy) between particles in a

The use of heterogenous catalysts for industrial reactions

Different reactions have different catalysts. Some industrial catalysts (which you will meet later in this book, see pages 88–89) are shown in table below. A **heterogeneous catalyst** is a catalyst that is in a different state from the reactants.

> **Tip:** If you are asked to explain 'heterogeneous catalyst' in an exam, explain both words.

Reaction	Catalyst	Type of catalysis
Reaction of sulfur dioxide and oxygen in the Contact process (see page 89) to make sulfuric acid.	Vanadium(V) oxide (this is also referred to as vanadium pentoxide)	Heterogeneous – the vanadium oxide is solid and in a different state to the reactants, sulfur dioxide and oxygen, which are gases.
Reaction of nitrogen and hydrogen in the Haber process (see pages 88–89) to make ammonia.	Iron	Heterogeneous – the iron is solid and in a different state to the reactants, nitrogen and hydrogen, which are gases.
Reaction of oxygen with ammonia in the Ostwald process to make nitric acid.	Platinum-rhodium	Heterogeneous – the platinum-rhodium is a solid and in a different state to the reactants, ammonia and oxygen, which are gases.

Catalysts make industrial processes more economic. Many industrial processes rely on catalysts to:

- speed up reactions, producing a **greater yield** of product and reducing manufacturing costs.
- provide a pathway of lower activation energy, so **less energy** is required for molecules to react, saving energy costs.
- benefit the environment, as catalysts reduce the amount of energy needed for particles to react, so less fossil fuel is burnt and less carbon dioxide is released into the atmosphere.

Chemisorption

Most heterogeneous catalysts work by **chemisorption**. The chemisorption process works in the following way:

- One or more of the reactants are **adsorbed** on to the surface of the catalyst at active sites.
- This causes bonds to weaken in the reactant molecules so the reaction occurs and products form.
- The product molecules desorb and leave the active site available for a new set of reactants to attach and react.

> **Tip: Ad**sorption is where something sticks to the surface of a substance, it is different from **ab**sorption where a substance is taken into a structure.

Catalytic converters

Gaseous pollutants from a car can be removed by **catalytic converters** attached to exhausts. A catalytic converter has a honeycomb ceramic structure coated with a metal catalyst (such as **platinum** or **rhodium**), which uses less metal than a solid metal catalyst structure. This helps keeps cost down. The honeycomb structure provides a large surface area for the reactions to take place, which ensures a faster and more complete reaction. This is **heterogeneous** catalysis, as the **catalyst** (solid) and the **reactants** (exhaust gases) are in **different states**.

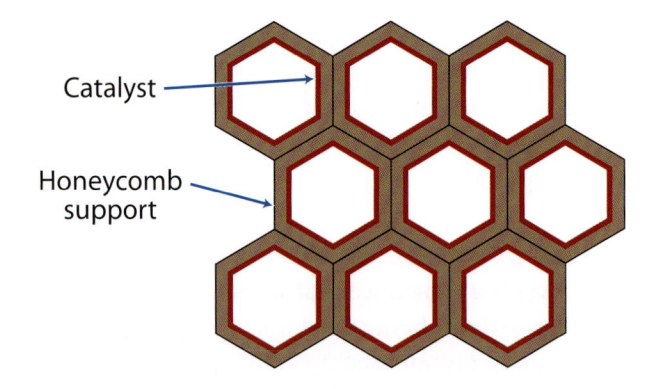

A catalytic converter

Exhaust gases such as carbon monoxide and nitrogen monoxide (NO) are converted to less-polluting products, such as carbon dioxide and nitrogen, by reactions on the surface of catalytic converters.

A catalyst has an active site that the reactant or substrate fits into to catalyse a reaction. Catalysts can be poisoned and made ineffective. In **catalytic**

3.4 KINETICS

Students should be able to:

3.4.1 define the terms rate of reaction and activation energy;

3.4.2 construct a reaction profile diagram;

3.4.3 explain the factors that affect the rate of a reaction, including concentration, pressure of gases, temperature and use of a catalyst;

3.4.4 explain common practical techniques to follow the rate of a reaction and analyse the effects of these factors;

3.4.5 demonstrate an understanding of collision theory;

3.4.6 recall and use the Maxwell-Boltzmann distribution curve to explain the effects of change in temperature and action of a catalyst on the rate of a given reaction;

3.4.7 describe the process of chemisorption in catalysis;

3.4.8 define the term catalyst and describe the role of a catalyst in a catalytic converter, including the concept of catalyst poisoning;

3.4.9 demonstrate an understanding of the use of a solid (heterogeneous) catalyst for industrial reactions; and

3.4.10 evaluate the economic benefits of using catalysts in industrial reactions, including the manufacture of ammonia, sulfuric acid and nitric acid.

Rate of reaction

The rate of a reaction is a measure of the speed at which reactants are changed into products.

In a fast reaction it takes a **short** time to convert reactants to products. Dynamite exploding and potassium reacting with water are examples of fast reactions. In a slow reaction it takes a **long** time to convert reactants to products. Rusting of iron is a slow reaction.

rate of reaction =

$$\frac{\text{quantity of reactant used or product formed}}{\text{time taken}}$$

> **Tip:** Reaction profiles for exothermic and endothermic reactions (as shown on pages 69–70) should also be revised for this topic.

Collision theory

Collision theory states that for a reaction to occur the reacting particles (these may be atoms, ions or molecules) must collide together with enough energy to react. **Activation energy (E_a) is the minimum energy needed for a reaction to occur.**

Successful collisions are ones that result in a reaction, and they take place when reactant particles collide with the activation energy. The activation energy is used to help break bonds so that the atoms can be rearranged to make products. Unsuccessful collisions are collisions that do not result in reaction and occur when the particles collide with less than the activation energy.

In general, reaction rates are increased when the frequency and energy of the collisions is increased.

> **Tip:** Frequency is the number of collisions in a certain amount of time.

Factors affecting the rate of reactions

Various factors can change the rate of a reaction, including:

1. Concentration of solution

Increasing the concentration of a solution increases the rate of reaction.

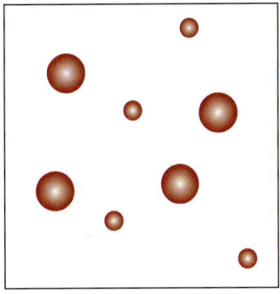

Low concentration   High concentration

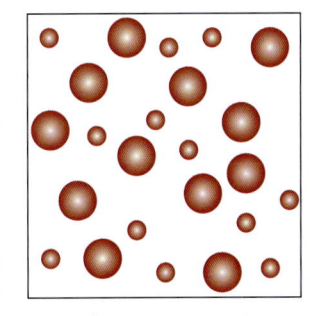

Explanation:
- There are more particles present in the same volume.
- This results in more successful collisions (with the activation energy) between particles in a

given time (the successful collisions are more frequent), and thus there is a faster rate of reaction.

2. Pressure of gases

Increasing the pressure of a gas increases the rate of reaction.

Explanation:
- The particles are pushed closer together.
- The same number of particles occupy a smaller volume.
- This results in more successful collisions (with the activation energy) between particles in a given time (the successful collisions are more frequent), and thus there is a faster rate of reaction.

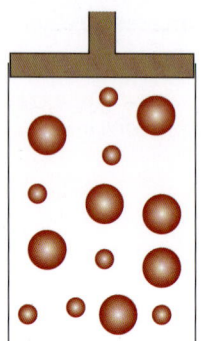

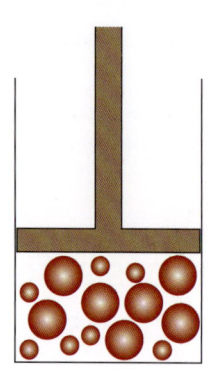

Low pressure   **Higher pressure**

3. Surface area of solid reactants

Increasing the surface area by breaking a solid reactant into smaller pieces increases the rate of reaction.

Explanation:
- There is a greater surface area so there are more particles on the surface exposed to the other reactant.
- This results in more successful collisions (with the activation energy) between particles in a given time (the successful collisions are more frequent), and thus there is a faster rate of reaction.

Tip: Remember that if a solid is broken up into smaller pieces, it has a bigger surface area.

4. Temperature

Increasing the temperature increases the rate of reaction.

Explanation:
- The particles are moving faster so there are more frequent collisions.
- The particles also have more energy so more of the particles have the activation energy and react when they collide.
- This results in more successful collisions between particles in a given time (the successful collisions are more frequent) and thus there is a faster rate of reaction.

In any system, the particles have a wide range of different energies. For **gases**, this can be shown on a graph called the **Maxwell-Boltzmann distribution curve**, which is a plot of the number of particles having each particular energy. The **most common energy** of the molecules is represented by the **peak** value and the **area under the curve** gives the **total number of particles**. The number of particles with energy greater than the activation energy (E_a) is shaded. Only the particles in this area of the graph have enough energy to react. To get more particles to react, the graph shape needs to change.

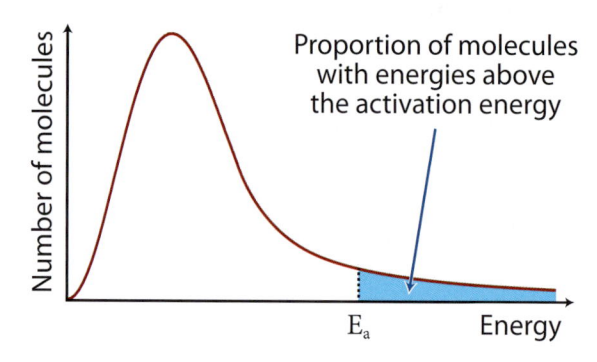

Maxwell-Boltzmann distribution curve

Tip: You will often be asked to sketch this graph – note that the line gets close to the *x*-axis but does not touch it.

Tip: Make sure you remember the correct labels for the axes for this graph.

3.4 KINETICS

A Maxwell-Boltzmann distribution curve can be used to explain the effects of change in temperature on the rate of a given reaction. The diagram below shows the distribution at a temperature (T_1) and a higher temperature (T_2). The total area under each graph is the same as the total number of reactant molecules is the same.

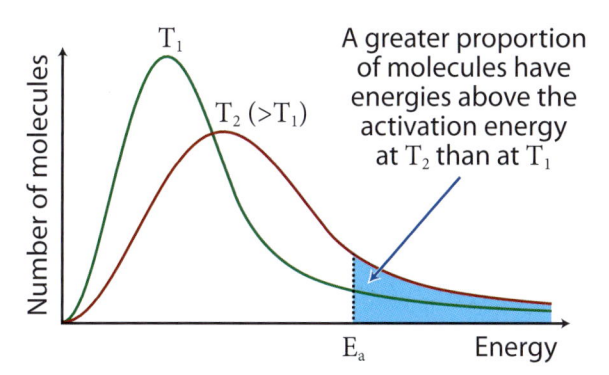

A Maxwell-Boltzmann distribution curve at different temperatures T_1 and T_2

When the temperature is increased:
- the peak value moves to the right.
- the peak is lower as the curve flattens slightly.

At the higher temperature, the reaction is faster (as the distribution shows).

- There are more molecules with greater energy than the activation energy (E_a), as shown by the **greater area** under the curve.
- This results in more successful collisions with the activation energy between particles in a given time (the successful collisions are more frequent), and thus there is a faster rate of reaction.

5. The presence of a catalyst
A catalyst is a substance that increases the rate of a reaction without being used up.

The catalyst is not used up in the reaction, so there should be the same mass the end of the reaction as at the start. As it is not used up, a catalyst should not appear in a chemical equation but may sometimes appear on top of the arrow.

A catalyst works in the following way:
- It provides a **different pathway** (route) of **lower** activation energy.
- As a result there are more particles with greater energy than the activation energy.

- This results in more successful collisions (with the activation energy) between particles in a given time (the successful collisions are more frequent), and thus there is a faster rate of reaction.

This is shown on the reaction profile below, which is for an exothermic reaction.

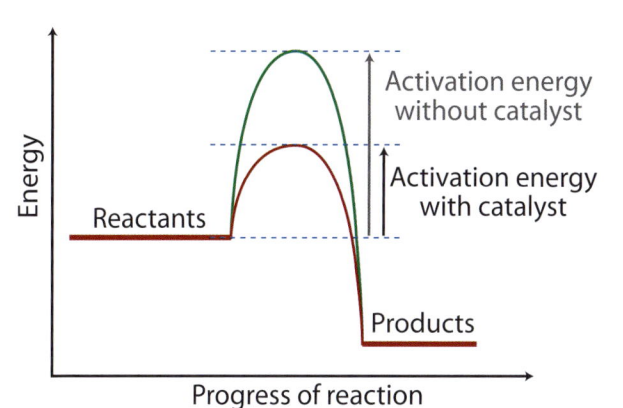

A reaction profile for a catalysed and uncatalysed reaction

> **Tip:** Always state that a catalyst provides a **different pathway** for the reaction, which has lower activation energy. It does not lower the activation energy.

A Maxwell-Boltzmann distribution curve can be used to explain the action of a catalyst on the rate of a given reaction. A catalyst provides a different pathway with lower activation energy. This means that more molecules have greater energy than the activation energy, as shown by the greater area under the distribution curve. This results in more successful collisions (with the activation energy) between particles in a given time, and thus there is a faster rate of reaction.

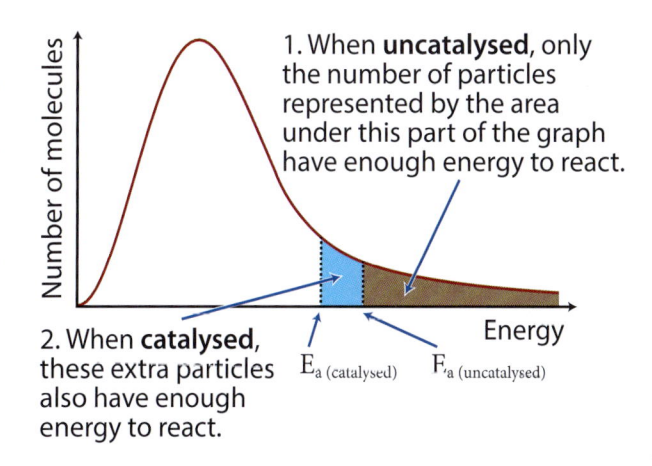

Maxwell-Boltzmann distribution curve to explain the effect of a catalyst on rate

81

The use of heterogenous catalysts for industrial reactions

Different reactions have different catalysts. Some industrial catalysts (which you will meet later in this book, see pages 88–89) are shown in table below. A **heterogeneous catalyst** is a catalyst that is in a different state from the reactants.

> **Tip:** If you are asked to explain 'heterogeneous catalyst' in an exam, explain both words.

Reaction	Catalyst	Type of catalysis
Reaction of sulfur dioxide and oxygen in the Contact process (see page 89) to make sulfuric acid.	Vanadium(V) oxide (this is also referred to as vanadium pentoxide)	Heterogeneous – the vanadium oxide is solid and in a different state to the reactants, sulfur dioxide and oxygen, which are gases.
Reaction of nitrogen and hydrogen in the Haber process (see pages 88–89) to make ammonia.	Iron	Heterogeneous – the iron is solid and in a different state to the reactants, nitrogen and hydrogen, which are gases.
Reaction of oxygen with ammonia in the Ostwald process to make nitric acid.	Platinum-rhodium	Heterogeneous – the platinum-rhodium is a solid and in a different state to the reactants, ammonia and oxygen, which are gases.

Catalysts make industrial processes more economic. Many industrial processes rely on catalysts to:

- speed up reactions, producing a **greater yield** of product and reducing manufacturing costs.
- provide a pathway of lower activation energy, so **less energy** is required for molecules to react, saving energy costs.
- benefit the environment, as catalysts reduce the amount of energy needed for particles to react, so less fossil fuel is burnt and less carbon dioxide is released into the atmosphere.

Chemisorption

Most heterogeneous catalysts work by **chemisorption**. The chemisorption process works in the following way:

- One or more of the reactants are **adsorbed** on to the surface of the catalyst at active sites.
- This causes bonds to weaken in the reactant molecules so the reaction occurs and products form.
- The product molecules desorb and leave the active site available for a new set of reactants to attach and react.

> **Tip:** **Ad**sorption is where something sticks to the surface of a substance, it is different from **ab**sorption where a substance is taken into a structure.

Catalytic converters

Gaseous pollutants from a car can be removed by **catalytic converters** attached to exhausts. A catalytic converter has a honeycomb ceramic structure coated with a metal catalyst (such as **platinum** or **rhodium**), which uses less metal than a solid metal catalyst structure. This helps keeps cost down. The honeycomb structure provides a large surface area for the reactions to take place, which ensures a faster and more complete reaction. This is **heterogeneous** catalysis, as the **catalyst** (solid) and the **reactants** (exhaust gases) are in **different states**.

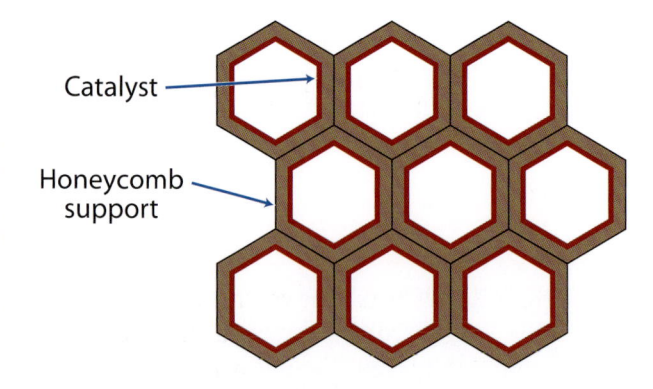

A catalytic converter

Exhaust gases such as carbon monoxide and nitrogen monoxide (NO) are converted to less-polluting products, such as carbon dioxide and nitrogen, by reactions on the surface of catalytic converters.

A catalyst has an active site that the reactant or substrate fits into to catalyse a reaction. Catalysts can be poisoned and made ineffective. In **catalytic**

poisoning, a substance that is not part of the reaction adsorbs to the catalyst's active sites. This blocks the active site, preventing reactants adsorbing and so deactivating the catalyst. For example, lead was once used in petrol. However, the lead poisons the catalyst in the catalytic converter by bonding to the active site, which stops the catalyst from working.

Common practical techniques to measure reaction rate

1. Measuring the volume of gas produced per unit time

If a reaction produces a gas, then the rate of reaction can be studied using the apparatus shown below. Examples of reactions that produce a gas include reaction of an acid and metal or acid and carbonate.

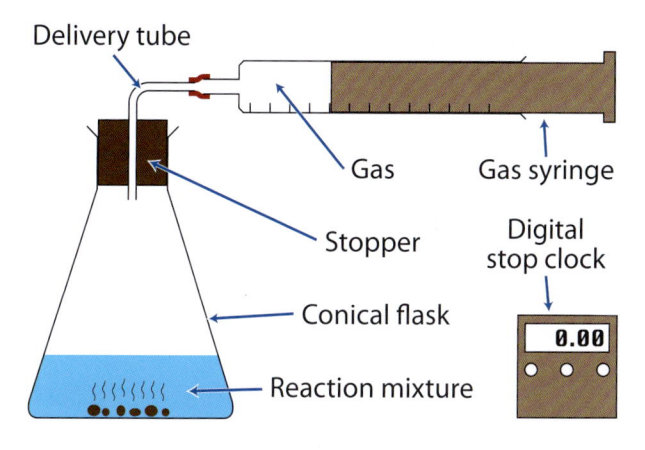

Investigating rate of reaction by measuring the volume of a gas produced

Tip: The stopper should be inserted quickly to ensure that no gas escapes when the solid reactant is added.

A stop clock is started and the volume of gas collected in the gas syringe recorded at various time intervals. The reaction is finished when two readings are the same, showing that no more gas is produced because one of the reactants is used up.

Tip: In a reaction, one of the two reactants is usually in excess – this means that it is not all used up and some is left at the end of the experiment. When one reactant is used up, the reaction is over.

A graph of volume of gas against time can be plotted. The gradient gives the rate. To study the effect of a variable such as concentration or temperature on rate, this variable can be changed and the experiment repeated to determine its effect on rate of reaction.

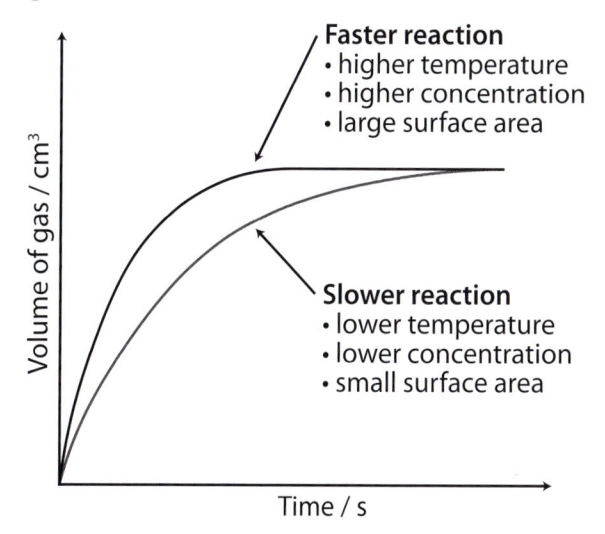

Graph of volume against time

Tip: Note that the faster reaction has a steeper gradient. The reactions both finish at the same time as the same amounts of reactants are used.

2. Measuring the change in mass in a given time

The change in mass during a reaction can be recorded at various time intervals using the apparatus shown below. If the reaction produces a gas, then the mass decreases because the gas escapes from the flask into the atmosphere. The cotton wool plug allows the gas out and prevents any liquid loss from the flask, as bubbling in the reaction may cause the solution to splash out.

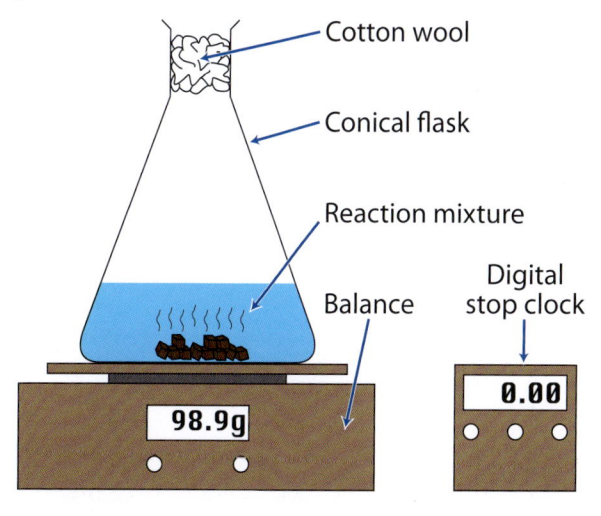

Investigating rate of reaction by measuring the change in mass in a given time

Tip: A graph of loss in mass against time, or simply mass against time (as shown here), can be plotted.

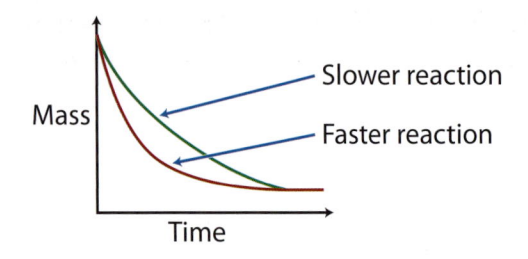

Questions

1. Define the terms:
   (a) rate of reaction [1]
   (b) activation energy [1] **[2 marks]**

2. Explain why the reaction of 0.2 g of magnesium with 25.0 cm³ of 2.0 mol dm⁻³ hydrochloric acid is faster than the reaction of 0.2 g of magnesium with 25.0 cm³ of 1.0 mol dm⁻³ hydrochloric acid. [2] **[2 marks]**

3. Explain if 1 g of calcium carbonate powder or 1 g of calcium carbonate chips will react faster with acid. [2] **[2 marks]**

4. (a) Using the letters A, B, C or D, identify the following on the diagram below:
   (i) enthalpy change [1]
   (ii) activation energy of the catalysed reaction [1]
   (iii) activation energy of the uncatalysed reaction [1]

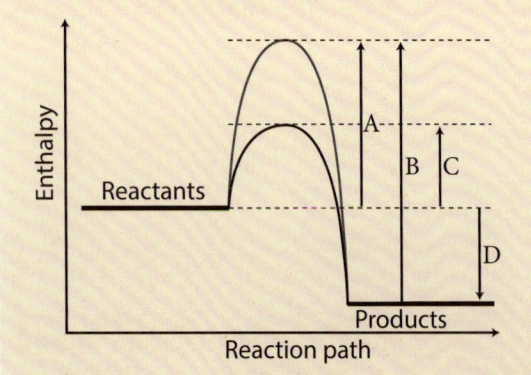

   (b) Explain if this is an exothermic reaction or endothermic reaction. [2] **[5 marks]**

5. (a) Define the term catalyst. [2]
   (b) Explain why a catalyst increases the rate of a reaction. [3]
   (c) Explain the term heterogeneous catalysis as applied to a catalytic converter. [2]
   (d) Explain why leaded petrol must not be used in cars fitted with a catalytic converter. [2]
   (e) Suggest why a honeycomb structure is used in the design of a catalytic converter. [1]
   (f) Explain the term chemisorption. [3]
   (g) Name the catalyst used in:
      (i) the Haber process [1]
      (ii) the production of nitric acid [1]
   [15 marks]

6. (a) Use the idea of activation energy to explain why an increase in temperature increases the rate of a reaction. [3]
   (b) State what happens to a Maxwell-Boltzmann curve if the temperature is increased. [2] **[5 marks]**

7. To study the rate of the reaction between calcium carbonate and hydrochloric acid, an experiment was carried out at room temperature and the volume of gas produced over time was measured.
   (a) List the apparatus used in this experiment. [3]
   (b) The experiment was repeated at a higher temperature to determine the effect of temperature on rate. How would you ensure this was a fair test? [2]
   (c) Compare the graph of volume of gas produced against time, in the two experiments. [2]
   (d) Use the idea of activation energy to explain why a decrease in temperature decreases the rate of a chemical reaction. [3]
   [10 marks]

3.5 EQUILIBRIUM

> **Students should be able to:**
>
> 3.5.1 define the terms reversible reaction and dynamic equilibrium;
>
> 3.5.2 state Le Châtelier's principle and use it to describe the qualitative effects of changes of conditions (temperature, pressure, concentration and catalysts) on the position of equilibrium for a closed homogeneous system;
>
> 3.5.3 recall the conditions and chemical equations required in the Haber process and Contact process; and
>
> 3.5.4 evaluate data to explain the need to reach a compromise between yield and rate of reaction for many industrial processes.

Reversible reactions

A reversible reaction is one in which the products, once made, can react to reform the reactants.

Reversible arrows ($\rightleftharpoons$) are used to show that a reaction is reversible. An example of a reversible reaction is the Haber process: $N_2 + 3H_2 \rightleftharpoons 2NH_3$ (see pages 88–89).

If a reversible reaction is exothermic in one direction and gives out heat, then it is endothermic in the other direction and takes in heat. The amount of energy transferred will be the same in each direction. For example, the reaction above gives out −92 kJ of energy in the forward reaction and the reverse reaction will take in +92 kJ of energy.

Dynamic equilibrium

A **closed system** is one in which no substances can get in or out (e.g. a test tube or a flask containing water with a stopper inserted is a closed system). An open system allows entry and exit of substances, for example an open beaker of boiling water. Reversible reactions can reach equilibrium in a closed system, when the rate of the forward and reverse reaction is equal and so the concentrations of reactants and products do not change.

When a system is in equilibrium there is no observable change but the system is in constant motion (**dynamic**). As fast as reactants are turned into products, the products are being turned back into reactants. Although nothing seems to be happening, the reaction is still taking place in both directions. All the species in the system are present.

Dynamic equilibrium occurs in a closed system when the rates of forward and reverse reactions are equal and the amounts/concentration of reactants and products remain constant.

The effects of changes of temperature, pressure and concentration on the position of equilibrium

At equilibrium, the relative amounts of reactants and products present depends on the conditions. If there are more products than reactants, we say the position of equilibrium is to the right-hand side. If there are more reactants than products, we say that the position of equilibrium is to the left. If there is a similar amount of reactants and products, the equilibrium position is in the middle.

If the conditions of a homogeneous reaction (temperature, pressure or concentration) are changed, then the position of equilibrium changes and so does the relative amounts of reactants and products.

> **Tip:** A homogeneous reaction is one in which the reactants and products are in the same phase.

Le Châtelier's principle

Le Châtelier's principle can be used to predict how changes in condition affect the position of equilibrium. It states that **if a change is made to the conditions of a system at equilibrium, then the position of the equilibrium moves to oppose that change in conditions.**

1. The effect of changing the concentration

If the concentration of a reactant or product in equilibrium (in a closed system) is changed, according to Le Châtelier's principle, the position of equilibrium will move to oppose the change. This means it will try to undo the effects of the change:

- if more of a chemical is added, the equilibrium position moves to remove it.
- if some of a chemical is removed, the equilibrium position moves to make more of it.

The table below summarises how changes in concentration affect the position of an equilibrium of the form: **reactants ⇌ products**

Changes in concentration	Effect on equilibrium position
Increase in concentration of a reactant	Moves right to reduce concentration of reactant
Decrease in concentration of a reactant	Moves left to increase concentration of reactant
Increase in concentration of a product	Moves left to reduce concentration of product
Decrease in concentration of a product	Moves right to increase concentration of product

Worked example

For the reaction, at constant temperature and pressure:

$$N_2 + 3H_2 \rightleftharpoons 2NH_3 \quad \Delta H = -92 \text{ kJ mol}^{-1}$$

state and explain what will happen to the amount of ammonia formed if:
(a) the concentration of nitrogen is increased.
(b) the ammonia is removed as soon as it is produced.

Answer
(a) If the concentration of nitrogen is increased:
- the equilibrium position moves right to reduce the concentration of added nitrogen.
- more ammonia is produced because the equilibrium position moves right.

(b) If the ammonia is removed, the concentration of ammonia decreases and:
- the equilibrium position moves right to increase the concentration of ammonia.
- more ammonia is produced because the equilibrium position moves right.

2. The effect of changing the temperature

If the temperature of an equilibrium reaction in a closed system is changed, according to Le Châtelier's principle, the position of equilibrium will move to oppose the change. This means it will move to undo the effects of the change:

- in order to increase the temperature, the equilibrium position moves in the exothermic direction.
- in order to decrease the temperature, the equilibrium position moves in the endothermic direction.

The table below summarises how changes in temperature affect the position of equilibrium for a reaction where the forward reaction is exothermic.

Change in temperature	Effect on equilibrium position	
	for a reaction where the forward reaction is exothermic	for a reaction where the forward reaction is endothermic
Increase in temperature	Moves left in endothermic direction to decrease the temperature	Moves right in endothermic direction to decrease the temperature
Decrease in temperature	Moves right in exothermic direction to increase the temperature	Moves left in exothermic direction to increase the temperature

Reactions that produce more product at **lower** temperatures are not usually carried out at low temperature. This is because they would be far too slow. A **compromise** temperature is often chosen, which balances a reasonable yield of product and a reasonable rate.

3.5 EQUILIBRIUM

Worked example
For the reaction:

$N_2 + 3H_2 \rightleftharpoons 2NH_3 \quad \Delta H = -92 \text{ kJ mol}^{-1}$

state and explain what happens to the amount of ammonia formed if the temperature is increased.

Tip: A negative ΔH value means the reaction is exothermic in the forward direction.

Answer
If the temperature is increased:
- the forward reaction is exothermic and the position of equilibrium moves left in the endothermic direction to reduce the temperature.
- less ammonia is produced because the equilibrium position moves left.

Worked example
Hydrogen can be made by reacting methane with steam.

$CH_{4(g)} + H_2O_{(g)} \rightleftharpoons 3H_{2(g)} + CO_{(g)}$

$\Delta H = +206.2 \text{ kJ mol}^{-1}$

State and explain the effect on the amount of hydrogen formed if the temperature is increased.

Answer
If the temperature is increased:
- the forward reaction is endothermic and the position of equilibrium moves right in the endothermic direction to reduce the temperature.
- more hydrogen is produced because the equilibrium position moves right.

3. The effect of changing the pressure

The more molecules that are present in a gas, the greater the pressure of the gas.

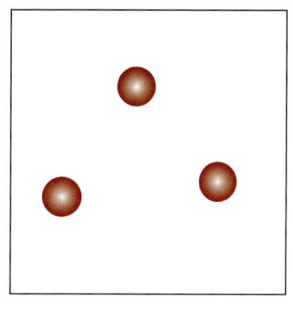

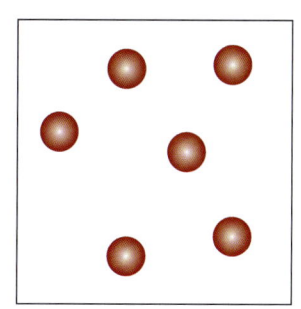

Lower pressure   Higher pressure

If the pressure of an equilibrium reaction in a closed system is changed, according to Le Châtelier's principle the position of equilibrium will move to oppose the change. This means it will move to undo the effects of the change:

- in order to increase the pressure, the equilibrium position moves to the side with the most gas molecules.
- in order to decrease the pressure, the equilibrium position moves to the side with the fewest gas molecules.

To determine the affect of pressure on the position of equilibrium it is important to first note down the total number of molecules on both sides of the equation. The table below shows how changes in pressure affect the position of equilibrium for three different reactions.

Reaction	Change in pressure	Effect on position of equilibrium
2A(g) ⇌ **B(g)** 2 molecules 1 molecule	Increase in pressure	Moves **right**, to the side with the fewest molecules, to decrease the pressure
	Decrease in pressure	Moves **left**, to the side with the most molecules, to increase the pressure
A(g) ⇌ **B(g)** 1 molecule 1 molecule	Increase in pressure	**Does not move** as there are the same number of gas molecules on each side of the equation
	Decrease in pressure	
A(g) + B(g) ⇌ **4 C(g)** 2 molecules 4 molecules	Increase in pressure	Moves **left**, to the side with the fewest molecules, to decrease the pressure
	Decrease in pressure	Moves **right**, to the side with more molecules, to increase the pressure

The use of high pressure is very expensive due to:
- the high cost of thick pipes to withstand the pressure.
- the high energy cost in compressing the gases.

In reactions where higher pressure gives more product, the value of the extra product formed is sometimes less than the cost of creating the higher pressure. This means that sometimes the actual pressure used in a process is not as high as might be predicted because it is not cost effective. There is often a **compromise** found between the amount of product formed and the cost of using higher pressure.

Worked example
In the equilibrium reaction:

nitrogen + hydrogen ⇌ ammonia
$N_2 + 3H_2 \rightleftharpoons 2NH_3$

state and explain what happens to the amount of ammonia formed if the pressure is increased at constant temperature.

Answer
nitrogen + hydrogen ⇌ ammonia
$N_{2(g)} + 3H_{2(g)} \rightleftharpoons 2NH_{3(g)}$

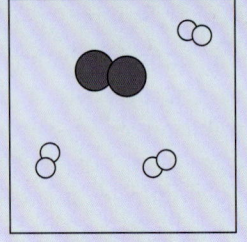

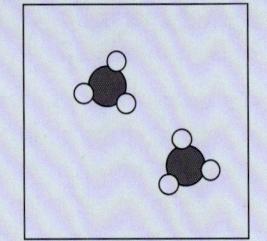

4 molecules: more pressure ⇌ 2 molecules: less pressure

If the pressure is increased:
- the equilibrium position moves right, to the side with fewer gas molecules, to decrease the pressure.
- more ammonia is produced because the equilibrium position moves right.

Tip: It is useful to draw out a quick diagram to show the number of molecules on each side; this will help your understanding. It is sufficient to represent all molecules with circles.

Worked example
Hydrogen can be made by reacting methane with steam.

$CH_{4(g)} + H_2O_{(g)} \rightleftharpoons 3H_{2(g)} + CO_{(g)}$

State and explain what happens to the amount of hydrogen formed if the pressure is increased at constant temperature.

Answer
methane + steam ⇌ hydrogen + carbon dioxide
$CH_{4(g)} + H_2O_{(g)} \rightleftharpoons 3H_{2(g)} + CO_{(g)}$

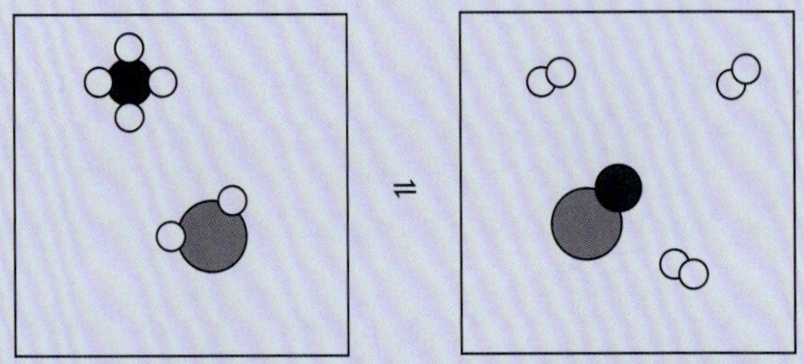

2 molecules: less pressure ⇌ 4 molecules: more pressure

If the pressure is increased:
- the equilibrium position moves left, to the side with fewer gas molecules, to decrease the pressure.
- less hydrogen is produced because the equilibrium position moves left.

4. The effect of adding a catalyst
A catalyst does not change the position of equilibrium, it simply speeds up the rate of a reaction. The catalyst speeds up the forward and the backward reaction by the same amount, which means it does not affect the relative rate of the two reactions or the position of equilibrium. Adding a catalyst speeds up only the rate at which a reaction reaches equilibrium.

Industrial examples of equilibrium reactions

1. The Haber process to produce ammonia
In industry, nitrogen and hydrogen react in an **exothermic** reaction to produce ammonia in the Haber process.

nitrogen + hydrogen ⇌ ammonia
$N_{2(g)} + 3H_{2(g)} \rightleftharpoons 2NH_{3(g)}$

What conditions give a high yield of ammonia?

(a) Temperature

Ammonia is produced by the forward exothermic reaction. **Decreasing** the temperature means that the position of equilibrium moves right in the exothermic direction to reduce the temperature and so producing more ammonia. However, although a low temperature produces a high yield, the reaction is too slow, so a **compromise** temperature of 450°C is used to give a reasonable rate of production and a reasonable yield.

(b) Pressure

If a **high** pressure is used, the equilibrium position moves right, to the side with fewer gas molecules, to decrease the pressure and more ammonia is produced. However, large amounts of energy are needed to compress the gases and the thick pipes needed to do this are expensive, so a **compromise** pressure of 200 atmospheres (atm) is used.

The conditions used in industry are:

- **temperature of 450°C**
- **pressure of 200 atm**
- **catalyst of iron**

A catalyst has no effect on the position of equilibrium, it simply speeds up the rate of reaction.

> **Tip:** Make sure you learn the conditions and equation for the Haber process.

2. The Contact process to produce sulfuric acid

There are three stages to the process to produce sulfuric acid:

Stage 1: Burning sulfur in air to form sulfur dioxide.

$$S_{(s)} + O_{2(g)} \rightarrow SO_{2(g)}$$

Stage 2: Reacting sulfur dioxide with more air in a reversible, exothermic reaction to produce sulfur trioxide. A catalyst of vanadium (V) oxide (vanadium pentoxide) is used in this stage.

$$2SO_{2(g)} + O_{2(g)} \rightleftharpoons 2SO_{3(g)}$$

Stage 3: The sulphur trioxide cannot be dissolved directly in water as it causes a **mist of corrosive fumes**. It is dissolved into concentrated (98%) sulfuric acid to form **oleum**, which is very concentrated sulfuric acid. Oleum is then diluted.

$$SO_3 + H_2SO_4 \rightarrow H_2S_2O_7$$
$$\text{(oleum)}$$
$$H_2S_2O_7 + H_2O \rightarrow 2H_2SO_4$$

Stage 2 is a reversible reaction and so the yield of product depends on the conditions used.

What conditions give a high yield of sulfur trioxide?

(a) Temperature

Sulfur trioxide is produced by the forward exothermic reaction. **Decreasing** the temperature means that the position of equilibrium moves right in the exothermic direction to reduce the temperature and so producing more sulfur trioxide. However, although a low temperature produces a high yield, the reaction is too slow, so a compromise temperature of 450°C is used to give a reasonable rate of production and a reasonable yield.

(b) Pressure

If a **high** pressure is used the equilibrium position moves right, to the side with fewer gas molecules (3 molecules on the left and 2 on the right), to decrease the pressure and more sulfur trioxide is produced. However, large amounts of energy is needed to compress the gases and the thick pipes needed to do this are expensive, so a compromise pressure of 1–2 atm is used. Even at this relatively low pressure, there is a 99.5% conversion of sulphur dioxide into sulphur trioxide, so the improvement in yield by increasing the pressure is not worth the expense in this case.

The conditions used in industry are:

- **temperature of 450°C**
- **pressure of 1–2 atm**
- **catalyst of vanadium(V) oxide**

> **Tip:** Make sure you learn the conditions and equation for the Contact process.

Questions

1. Define the terms:
   (a) reversible reaction [1]
   (b) dynamic equilibrium [2]   [3 marks]

2. Complete the table below for the Haber and Contact processes.   [10 marks]

	Haber process	Contact process
Symbol equation		
Temperature (°C)		
Pressure (atm)		
Catalyst		

3. For the reaction:
   $2NO_{(g)} + O_{2(g)} \rightleftharpoons 2NO_{2(g)}$
   $\Delta H = -116$ kJ mol^{-1}

   State and explain the effect of increasing:
   (a) the pressure [2]
   (b) the temperature [2]
   on the position of equilibrium.   [4 marks]

4. Methanol is made in industry by the reaction below:
   $CO_{2(g)} + 3H_{2(g)} \rightleftharpoons CH_3OH_{(g)} + H_2O_{(g)}$
   $\Delta H = -49$ kJ mol^{-1}

   (a) Explain if high or low pressure would give a maximum equilibrium yield of methanol. [2]
   (b) Explain why the actual pressure used by the chemical industry might be different. [1]
   (c) Explain if high or low temperature would give a maximum equilibrium yield of methanol. [2]
   (d) Explain why the actual temperature used by the chemical industry might be different. [1]   [6 marks]

5. For the preparation of propenenitrile (CH_2CHCN), the conditions used are 450°C and 2.5 atmospheres.
   $C_3H_6 + NH_3 + 1½O_2 \rightleftharpoons CH_2CHCN + 3H_2O$
   $\Delta H = -540$ kJ mol^{-1}

   Describe and explain the effect on the position of equilibrium of:
   (a) a temperature above 450°C [2]
   (b) a pressure above 2.5 atmospheres. [2]   [4 marks]

6. What condition is required for a dynamic equilibrium to be established?   [1 mark]

3.6 INDUSTRIAL PROCESSES

Students should be able to:

3.6.1 explain the terms batch and continuous process;

3.6.2 demonstrate an understanding that industry must take into account capital, direct and indirect costs when manufacturing chemicals on a large scale;

3.6.3 compare and contrast the differences between industrial-scale and laboratory-scale production of chemicals;

3.6.4 demonstrate an understanding of the economics linked to scaling up a laboratory reaction;

3.6.5 demonstrate an understanding of the link between production costs and determining the selling price of a chemical; and

3.6.6 consider the impact of factors such as: waste management, infrastructure and environmental consequences on the choice of site for a new chemical manufacturing plant.

Batch and continuous processes in industry

Chemicals can be manufactured in industry from raw materials in their unprocessed state by a continuous process or a batch process.

A continuous process is a non-stop process where products are removed at the same time as new reactants are added.

A continuous process is used to manufacture **large amounts** of chemicals. It is usually a partially automated process, needing small numbers of employees, which keeps labour costs low. A continuous process is carried out in a dedicated manufacturing plant, designed to produce one product, with reactants being fed in and products being removed continuously.

Examples of continuous processes include:
- the Haber process to manufacture ammonia.
- the Contact process to manufacture sulfuric acid.
- fractional distillation of crude oil.
- fertiliser manufacture.

Advantages of a continuous process include:
- it generally has a fast rate of production.
- it is often a partially automated process, not labour intensive and so labour costs are low.
- it can produce large amounts of the chemical.

Disadvantages of a continuous process include:
- high capital costs, as plant set up costs are high.
- it is specific for one chemical or product.
- it can have very complex control systems, so if any part of the technology breaks down the plant may need to stop running, which is costly.
- poor accessibility for maintenance or repair, due to the large size of the plant.

A batch process is an intermittent process where reactants are added, a reaction occurs and products are removed. The vessel is then cleaned and the process started again with new reactants.

A batch process is used when a chemical is needed in a **small amount** (e.g. when trialling a process to manufacture a chemical or when a speciality chemical, such as a specific medicine, is needed). The equipment is assembled for the reaction needed, rather than using a plant of equipment dedicated to one process.

Examples of where batch processes are used include:
- in research laboratories, during the early stages of developing processes to manufacture chemicals.
- in processes where the product being made needs to change, such as pharmaceutical drug manufacture.
- in food manufacture, as it is easier to make slight variations to the process.

Advantages of a batch process include:
- it has low set up and plant costs (low capital costs), so it is useful for manufacturing small quantities (e.g. in research).
- it is a flexible process, which is not specific to one chemical or product. This makes it easy to make slight variations in products from batch to batch.

- it has simple control systems and low technology, making it easy to adjust.
- there is good accessibility for maintenance, due to the smaller size of the equipment.

Disadvantages of a batch process include:
- it is less automated, so more labour intensive, with higher labour costs.
- it needs cleaned and started up again between every batch, which is labour intensive and slows down the process.

The table below compares aspects of continuous and batch processes.

	Continuous	Batch
cost of factory equipment	high	low
shut down times	rare	often
labour costs	low	high
rate of production	high	low
automation	very automated	not as automated

Tip: You may be asked to compare advantages and disadvantages of a batch or continuous process. This table should help.

Industrial costs

Industry must take into account capital, direct and indirect costs when manufacturing chemicals on a large scale.

Capital cost is the cost of setting up a business or plant. In general, it is a 'one off' cost.

Examples of capital costs include:
- construction of the plant
- plant equipment
- storage for raw materials
- design fees

Tip: Remember that a raw material is an unprocessed material from which a product is made.

Indirect cost means that the cost per unit of the product is not directly proportional to this cost. Indirect costs stay the same at all levels of output and are related to maintenance, research and office work.

Examples of indirect costs include:
- insurance of the plant
- rent of the plant
- sales and marketing
- maintenance of the plant
- research and development
- labour

Direct cost means the cost per unit of the product is directly proportional to this cost. Direct costs are ongoing costs to run the process. If the manufacturer does not produce anything then the direct costs are zero.

Examples of direct costs include:
- fuel
- electricity
- raw materials (reactants and catalysts)
- packaging
- transport

The production cost of a chemical includes capital, indirect and direct costs. There is a strong link between the production cost and the selling price of a chemical. If the production costs are high, the selling price of a chemical must be high for the industry to make a suitable profit. The selling price will also depend on the demand for the product. Manufacturers carry out research and development to look at the different starting materials, reaction sequences and processing methods that can be used to make a chemical before deciding on a method of production. They do this to decide which method is most economic.

Sometimes, during a process, a by-product is produced in a side reaction. In most cases it is best to minimise by-product production as it complicates the process and must be isolated. However, if the by-product can be sold for a profit, this can lower production costs and lead to a higher profit. If energy is generated during the process then the excess energy can also be sold.

Tip: Make sure you learn definitions of each type of cost and are able to give examples.

Differences between industrial-scale and laboratory-scale production of chemicals

Only small quantities of chemicals can be produced in the laboratory. In industry, much larger quantities are manufactured. However, scaling up to industrial scale presents various problems (see table below). In the laboratory, small masses of chemicals can be weighed on a balance and quickly added to a flask. In industry, tonnes of chemicals need to be weighed out using specialist equipment and reaction vessels big enough to hold them need to be designed.

Choosing a site for a new chemical manufacturing plant

A new chemical manufacturing plant can bring various benefits to the local community:

- It generates money for the local economy, as commuting employees bring trade to local shops and businesses.
- It improves infrastructure and services, as good transport links (road and rail) and services (water, gas, electricity and Internet) are needed.
- It creates various employment opportunities for specialist staff (such as scientists, researchers and engineers) and support staff (such as clerical, canteen and security staff).

However, the impacts of various factors must be considered when choosing a site for a new plant.

1. Environmental consequences

Chemical manufacture is unavoidably harmful to the environment and can impact it in various ways:

- **Air pollution** – chemical plants can emit harmful waste gases, such as sulfur dioxide, which can cause acid rain and respiratory problems for humans and wildlife.
- **Water pollution** – chemical plants can discharge hot water, resulting in thermal pollution (which reduces the dissolved oxygen content of lakes and rivers causing eutrophication).
- **Noise pollution** – chemical plants emit noise from the vehicles used to transport and transfer both the raw materials and finished product, and from the machinery used to manufacture the chemicals.
- **Depletion of resources** – many raw materials are taken from the earth, air and water, so finite resources are removed.

The choice of site can also be impacted in the following ways:

- A chemical plant should not be sited near a city, as it may produce air pollution and noise pollution, which could both affect the health and well-being of residents.
- A chemical plant should not be sited near an area of natural beauty because it is an eyesore and causes the loss of habitat for wildlife.

	Laboratory preparation	**Industrial production**
Materials	• Small quantities – cost is not a big issue. • Most chemicals are readily available.	• Larger quantities – cost will limit the choice of material used. • There may be a limited choice of chemicals, as some are not available in large amounts.
Reaction	• Normal laboratory conditions are used – no extreme temperatures or pressures. • Normal-sized reaction vessels are used.	• Higher temperatures and pressures are possible using specialised equipment. Sensors are included to monitor temperature and pressure. • Large, specially-designed reaction vessels are used. These often have automated stirrers and pipework to transfer the materials. Heating and cooling systems (e.g. heat exchangers) are often part of the equipment.
Waste disposal	• Small quantities are easily disposed of.	• Larger quantities pose a disposal problem, especially if the waste is harmful.

Differences between laboratory-scale and industrial-scale processes

2. Infrastructure

Infrastructure affects the choice of site in the following ways:

- It must be close to good road and rail links for transport of raw materials and distribution of the finished product.
- It must be close to a town or population to provide workers for the plant.
- It may need to be close to a source of the bulk raw material(s), as this reduces transport costs.

3. Waste management

In Northern Ireland, all planning applications for industrial plants must adhere to guidelines for waste management requirements as set out in 'Required Environmental Information: A guide to supporting information required for effective consultations' (Northern Ireland Environment Agency, April 2015). These guidelines ensure that, before planning permission is granted for a site, waste management requirements have been met and the following strategies are in place:

- Sufficient drainage and water treatment for the plant.
- Measures to control air pollution.
- Hazard regulations and safety factors to cope with major accident or chemical spillages.
- Measures to store and dispose of hazardous waste.

Questions

1. Fractional distillation is a process used to separate a crude oil mixture into diesel, petrol, kerosene and other fractions. Different costs are involved in the process.
   (a) Define the term capital cost and give one example. [2]
   (b) Identify two direct costs and two indirect costs of fractional distillation. [4]
   (c) Fractional distillation is a continuous process. Define the term continuous process. [1]
   (d) Some processes can be batch processes. Define the term batch process. [1]
   (e) A continuous process often costs less than a batch process. Give one other advantage of a continuous process compared to a batch process. [1]
   (f) What is a raw material? [1]   **[10 marks]**

2. State three effects on the environment that the construction of a new chemical manufacturing plant may have.   **[3 marks]**

3. For a chemical manufacturing plant, classify each of the following as a direct, indirect or capital cost.
   (a) Research and development [1]
   (b) Plant construction [1]
   (c) Electricity [1]
   (d) Insurance [1]
   (e) Transport of the product [1]   **[5 marks]**

Unit AS 5:
Material Science

5.1 MATERIAL PROPERTIES

Students should be able to:

5.1.1 investigate practically a range of materials to demonstrate an understanding of how they are selected depending on their properties;

5.1.2 define chemical resistance as the ability of a material to withstand chemical attack and know that the addition of other materials can increase chemical resistance, for example chromium to steel to make stainless steel;

5.1.3 recall and use the equation for electrical conductivity, σ:

$$\text{conductivity } (\sigma) = \frac{\text{length } (L)}{\text{resistance } (R) \times \text{cross section area } (A)}$$

and know that electrical conductivity is measured in siemens per metre ($S\,m^{-1}$);

5.1.4 recall and use the equation for the rate of flow of heat, $\frac{Q}{t}$, through a material in the form of a bar of uniform cross section area A, length d and having a temperature difference ΔT across its ends, given by

$$\frac{Q}{t} = \frac{kA\Delta T}{d}$$

where k is the material's thermal conductivity and know that thermal conductivity is measured in $W\,m^{-1}\,°C^{-1}$;

5.1.5 recall and use the equation for the coefficient of friction, μ:

$$\text{coefficient of friction } (\mu) = \frac{\text{friction } (F)}{\text{normal reaction } (R)};$$

5.1.6 recall that the ductility of a material is a measure of its ability to be drawn into a wire and that most metals are ductile, but ceramics are not;

5.1.7 recall that malleability of a material is a measure of its ability to be hammered, pressed, or rolled into thin sheets without breaking, and that most metals are malleable, but ceramics are not;

5.1.8 recall that a material is showing elastic behaviour when it returns to its original dimensions following tension or compression;

5.1.9 recall that a material is showing plastic behaviour when it undergoes permanent deformation when in a state of tension or compression;

5.1.10 recall that tensile strength is the maximum stress that a material can withstand while being stretched or pulled before breaking and determine its value from a stress-strain graph;

5.1.11 recall that the yield strength is that stress at which elastic deformation ends and plastic deformation begins;

5.1.12 recall and use the equation for stress, σ

$$\text{stress } (\sigma) = \frac{\text{force } (F)}{\text{cross section area } (A)}$$

and know that stress in measured in pascals;

5.1.13 recall and use the equation for strain:

$$\text{strain } (\varepsilon) = \frac{\text{change in length } (\Delta L)}{\text{original length } (L_O)}$$

and know that strain has no units;

5.1.14 recall and use the equation for the Young modulus, E:

$$\text{Young modulus } (E) = \frac{\text{stress } (\sigma)}{\text{strain } (\varepsilon)}$$

and know that the Young modulus is measured in pascals;

5.1.15 conduct experiments to determine:
- stress, strain, and the Young modulus for the material of a metal wire;
- electrical conductivity of the material of a metal wire;

5.1.16 describe, in detail, the Vickers method to determine the hardness of a material and recall that the Vickers hardness number is measured in $N\,m^{-2}$;

5.1.17 interpret and draw conclusions about materials when presented with stress-strain graphs;

5.1.18 carry out and describe an experiment that will yield a stress-strain graph demonstrating plasticity;

5.1.19 demonstrate an understanding of the concepts of creep and fatigue strength;

5.1.20 recall and use the equation:

$$\text{density } (\rho) = \frac{\text{mass } (m)}{\text{volume } (V)}; \text{ and}$$

5.1.21 convert densities from non-common units for comparison purposes, for example comparing $g\,cm^{-3}$ to $kg\,l^{-1}$.

Mankind has used materials for thousands of years. For example, during the Stone Age, natural materials like stone, clay and wood were used. Useful materials such as bronze and iron were developed later. Even today, new materials are continually being developed to meet the needs of modern society.

Different materials have different properties due to their different chemical structure and bonding. These properties influence which materials are selected for different purposes. In this chapter, we shall explore the wide range of properties that materials can have.

Density

Density is the mass per unit volume of a substance. In a solid, the atoms or molecules fit closely together so the density is greater than that of a gaseous material, where the atoms or molecules are farther apart. Density has the symbol ρ and is represented by the equation:

$$\text{density } (\rho) = \frac{\text{mass } (m)}{\text{volume } (V)}$$

The common unit of density is $kg\ m^{-3}$. However, different units can be given, depending on the units the mass and the volume were measured in. For example, if the mass is measured in g and the volume in cm^3 then the unit of density is $g\ cm^{-3}$. If the mass is measured in kg and the volume is measured in litres ($1000\ cm^3$) then the unit of density is $kg\ l^{-1}$. You may need to convert densities from these non-common units in order to compare different measurements meaningfully.

Worked example
(a) Calculate the density, with units, of a metal cube that has a mass of 27 g and a volume of $5.0\ cm^3$.
(b) Convert your answer from part (a) to $kg\ m^{-3}$.

Answer
(a) $\text{density } (\rho) = \frac{\text{mass } (m)}{\text{volume } (V)}$

Tip: Always write down the equation you are using, when carrying out calculations.

$= \frac{27\ g}{5.0\ cm^3} = 5.4\ g\ cm^{-3}$

(b) $1\ kg = 1000\ g$, so $5.4\ g\ cm^{-3}$
$= 5.4 \div 1000$
$= 0.0054\ kg\ cm^{-3}$

$1\ m^3 = 1 \times 10^6\ cm^3$, so $0.0054\ kg\ cm^{-3}$
$= 0.0054 \times 1 \times 10^6$
$= 5.4 \times 10^3\ kg\ m^{-3}$

Tip: $1000\ cm^3 = 1\ dm^3$, and $1000\ dm^3 = 1\ m^3$.

Worked example
(a) What is the density of a board with dimensions $199\ cm \times 10.6\ cm \times 5.54\ cm$ and a mass of 28.6 kg? Give your answer in $g\ cm^{-3}$.
(b) The density of water is $1.0\ g\ cm^{-3}$. Suggest if the board will sink or float in water.

Answer
(a) The mass of the board is $28.6\ kg = 28600\ g$
The volume of the board is calculated using:
volume = length × breadth × height

$\text{density } (\rho) = \frac{\text{mass } (m)}{\text{volume } (V)}$

$= \frac{28600}{199 \times 10.6 \times 5.54}$

$= 2.45\ g\ cm^{-3}$ (to 3 s.f.)

Tip: The data in the question is given to three significant figures, so the answer is also given to three significant figures.

(b) Any substance with a density greater than $1.0\ g\ cm^{-3}$ will sink in water, so this board will sink.

Chemical resistance

Chemical resistance is the ability of a material to withstand chemical attack.

Chemical resistance is a measure of a material's resistance to corrosive environments. Some materials are not very chemically resistant. For example, iron is easily attacked by water and air to form **rust**.

Adding other materials can increase chemical resistance. For example, small amounts of chromium are added to steel to make **stainless steel**, which is more chemically resistant. Other materials, such as ceramics, are very chemically resistant. A sink, for example, must be made of a chemically resistant material such as ceramic, as it is regularly exposed to acids and alkalis.

Thermal conductivity

Thermal conductivity (k) is a measure of the ability of a material to conduct heat.

Thermal conductivity is measured in W m^{-1} °C^{-1} (watts per metre per degree Celsius). Some materials are better conductors of heat than others. Copper is a good thermal conductor and has thermal conductivity of 380 W m^{-1} °C^{-1} whereas air has a thermal conductivity of 0.025 W m^{-1} °C^{-1}. Gases have much lower thermal conductivity than solids because the atoms or molecules are farther apart and therefore do not transfer the heat energy between them as effectively.

The equation for rate of flow of heat through a bar of uniform cross section area A, length d with a temperature difference across its ends is given by:

Rate of flow of heat $= \dfrac{Q}{t} = \dfrac{kA\Delta T}{d}$

where: $\dfrac{Q}{t}$ = rate of flow of heat (W)

k = the material's thermal conductivity (W m^{-1} °C^{-1})

A = the cross section area of the bar (m^2)

ΔT = temperature difference between hot and cold sides (°C)

d = distance between hot and cold sides (m)

Worked example
Calculate the rate of heat transfer through a rectangular window on a cold day. The window is 1.2 m wide and 1.8 m high, has a thickness of 6.2 mm and a thermal conductivity of 0.27 W m^{-1} °C^{-1}. The temperature inside the home is 21°C and the temperature outside the home is 4°C.

Answer
Cross section area (area of window)
$A = 1.2 \times 1.8$ m = 2.16 m^2.
The distance (thickness of window) is given in mm and must be converted to metres by dividing by 10 to convert to cm and then by 100 to convert to m: d = 6.2 mm = 0.0062 m.
$\Delta T = 21 - 4 = 17$°C.

Rate of flow of heat
$= \dfrac{Q}{t} = \dfrac{kA\Delta T}{d} = \dfrac{0.27 \times 2.16 \times 17}{0.0062}$
$= 1599.10$ W ≈ 1600 W to 2 s.f.

Electrical conductivity

Electrical conductivity is a measure of the ability of a material to carry an electrical current.

An electric current is a flow of charge carriers through a material. Metals have high electrical conductivity because they have many delocalised electrons, which can move and carry charge. Electrical conductivity is measured in siemens per metre (S m^{-1}). It is defined by the equation:

conductivity (σ)
$= \dfrac{\text{length } (L)}{\text{resistance } (R) \times \text{cross section area } (A)}$
$= \dfrac{L}{RA}$

where: σ = conductivity (S m^{-1})
L = length of conductor (m)
R = resistance (Ω)
A = the cross section area (m^2)

Tip: You will learn more about metals conducting electricity, and their structure on page 110.

Experiment to measure electrical conductivity of the material of a metal wire

Method
- A resistance wire is straightened to ensure it does not have any bends or kinks. The diameter of the wire is measured at about five points along its length using a micrometer screw gauge and the average diameter calculated. The average cross section area of the wire is calculated using the equation for cross section area: $A = \frac{1}{4}\pi d^2$ where d is the average diameter of the wire.
- The resistance wire is secured along a metre stick using insulating tape.

Tip: A long piece of wire is used to get a measurable resistance.

- The remainder of the apparatus is set up as shown in the diagram overleaf, with one crocodile clip attached to the wire at the 'zero' end of the metre stick.

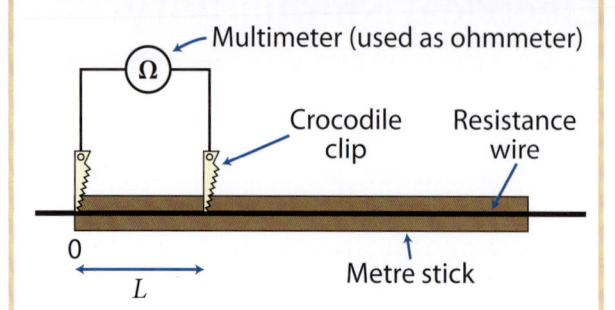

- The other crocodile clip is first placed at the 10 cm mark on the resistance wire and the resistance, R, read from the multimeter and recorded.
- The **length**, L, of the wire is then **increased** in steps of 10 cm by moving the second crocodile clip and recording the **resistance** for each length.
- The experiment is then repeated and the average resistance for each length of wire is calculated.
- The electrical conductivity is then calculated using the equation:

$$\sigma = \frac{L}{RA}$$

Tip: Remember that electrical conductivity is measured in siemens per metre ($S\ m^{-1}$).

Alternative Method

A similar experiment can be carried out using the circuit below.

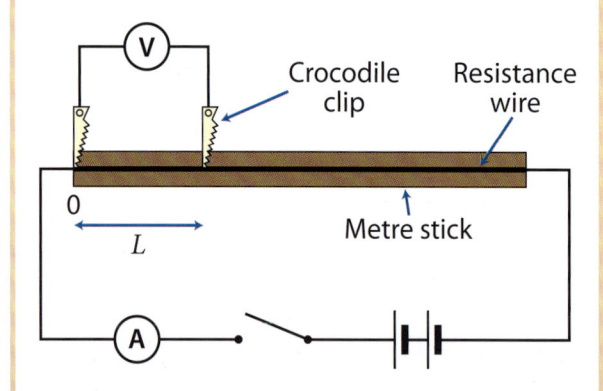

Instead of a multimeter, the current, I, through the wire is measured with an ammeter connected in series and the voltage across the wire, V, measured with a voltmeter. The resistance is calculated using $R = \frac{V}{I}$ and electrical conductivity calculated as above.

Tip: Remember that, to improve reliability and accuracy, the readings should be repeated and averaged; a long length of wire used; and the wire checked to ensure there are no kinks.

Worked example
What is the electrical conductivity of a wire of length 405 cm, a cross section area of $2.54 \times 10^{-8}\ m^2$ and a resistance of 2.50 Ω?

Answer
First write down the information in the question, using the correct units:
L = 4.05 m
A = $2.54 \times 10^{-8}\ m^2$
R = 2.50 Ω

Tip: If a length is given in cm or mm, make sure that you convert it to metres before using it in the equation (1 m = 100 cm = 1000 mm).

Then substitute the values into the equation for electrical conductivity:

$$\sigma = \frac{L}{RA} = \frac{4.05}{2.54 \times 10^{-8} \times 2.50}$$

$$= 63779527.56$$

$$= 6.38 \times 10^7\ S\ m^{-1}\ \text{(to 3 s.f.)}$$

Tip: In this question, the data is all given to 3 significant figures, so the answer can be given to 3 significant figures. It is best to do this using standard form.

Hardness

Hardness is a measure of how resistant a solid is to permanent shape change when a compressive force is applied.

In most tests for hardness, an object is pressed into the material to indent it, and the size of the dent is measured. The Vickers method outlined here involves measuring the length of a dent made by the impact of a diamond and can be used for all types of metals. The Vickers method gives very accurate readings. However, the machine required to carry out the test must be floor mounted and is very expensive.

5.1 MATERIAL PROPERTIES

Experiment to determine hardness ('Vickers method')

Method
- A square-based pyramid with a diamond tip is used to indent the material. There is an angle of 136° between opposite faces, as shown in the diagram. This gives an angle to the horizontal plane of 22° on each side of the pyramid.
- A force load of between 10 N and 1000 N (or between 1g and 100g, where g = acceleration due to gravity) is applied to the material for a time of 10–15 seconds.
- The lengths of the two diagonals of the indentation left in the surface of the material (d_1 and d_2) are measured and their average calculated. The area of the sloping surface of the indentation is then calculated.
- The force load is divided by the area of indentation to give the hardness.
- The unit of hardness given by the test is known as the Vickers hardness number (VHN). This is often converted to $N\ m^{-2}$.

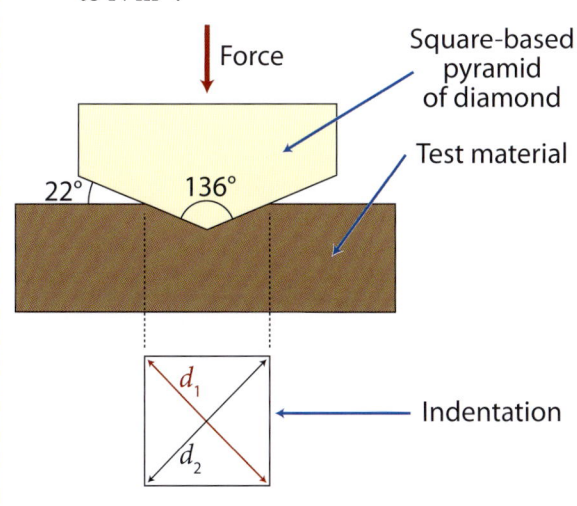

Malleability

Malleability is the measure of the ability of a material to be hammered, pressed or rolled into thin sheets without breaking.

Many metals are malleable. For example, copper can be hammered into sheets and used for a variety of purposes from saucepans to statues. Ceramics, by contrast, are not malleable and will tend to break if hammered or pressed.

The coefficient of friction

Friction is a force that resists motion when two objects are in contact. Different materials exert different amounts of frictional resistance. It is easier to drag an object over a sheet of glass than over sandpaper, because sandpaper exerts more frictional resistance than glass.

The level of friction that different materials exhibit is given by the **coefficient of friction (μ)**. The **coefficient of friction is the ratio of the force of friction between two bodies and the force pressing them together**. It is calculated using the equation:

$$\text{coefficient of friction } (\mu) = \frac{\text{friction force } (F)}{\text{normal reaction } (R)}$$

where: μ = coefficient of friction (no unit)
F = friction force (N)
R = normal reaction (N)

The normal reaction is the force with which one surface is being pushed into another. Usually the normal reaction is calculated using the equation:

$$F = mg$$

where: m = mass (kg)
g = acceleration due to gravity (9.8 $N\ kg^{-1}$)

For example, if a brick with a mass of 5 kg is lying on the ground, then the normal reaction is $5 \times 9.8 = 49$ N.

The coefficient of friction is dependent on both the material of the surface and the material of the body that is sliding over it. It provides a measure of the ease with which the surface of one material will slide over another material. Coefficients of friction range from near zero to greater than one. For example, ice moves quite freely across steel and has a low coefficient of friction, whereas rubber on a footpath has a high coefficient of friction.

Worked example
A body of mass 4 kg is placed on a horizontal plane. The frictional force when the body is just about to move is 10 N. Calculate the coefficient of friction between the body and the plane. The acceleration due to gravity is 9.8 N kg^{-1}.

Answer
Normal reaction, $R = mg = 4 \times 9.8 = 39.2$ N
Then using:

$$\text{coefficient of friction } (\mu) = \frac{\text{friction force } (F)}{\text{normal reaction } (R)}$$

$$= \frac{10}{39.2} = 0.26$$

Worked example
Calculate the stress in a wire of diameter 0.32 mm when a force of 4.50 N is applied to it.

Answer
First change the diameter from mm to metres. 1000 mm = 1 m, so divide by 1000:
$d = 0.32 \div 1000 = 0.00032$ or 3.2×10^{-4} m.
Then calculate the area using the equation:

$$A = \frac{\pi d^2}{4}$$

$$A = \frac{\pi d^2}{4} = \frac{\pi (0.00032)^2}{4} = \frac{3.22 \times 10^{-7}}{4}$$

$$= 8.05 \times 10^{-8}$$

Then calculate the stress using the equation:

$$\sigma = \frac{F}{A} = \frac{4.50}{8.05 \times 10^{-8}} = 5.6 \times 10^7 \text{ N m}^{-2}$$

Stress, strain and Young modulus

When a material is stretched, it becomes longer. We say that it has been put under tensile **stress** and as a result the material has become **strained**. A stiff material, such as iron, will not change its shape much when a strain is applied, but a soft material, such as clay, can be strained a lot, even with a small stress.

Stress
Stress (σ) is the applied force per unit cross section area. Stress is measured in pascals (Pa) or N m^{-2}. Stress can be calculated using the equation:

$$\text{Stress } (\sigma) = \frac{\text{force } (F)}{\text{cross section area } (A)}$$

where: σ = stress (Pa or N m^{-2})
F = force (N)
A = cross section area (m^2)

To work out the cross section area of a wire you may need to use the equation:

$$A = \frac{\pi d^2}{4}$$

where: d = the diameter of the wire (m)

or:

$$A = \pi r^2$$

where: r = the radius of the wire (m)

Strain

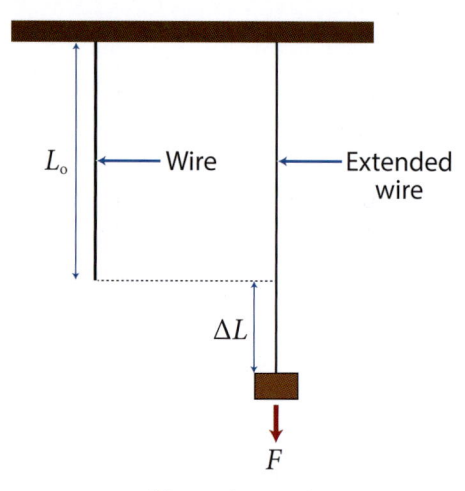

Measuring strain

Stress causes strain. **Strain (ε) is the extension (change in length) per unit length.** Strain can be calculated using the equation:

$$\text{Strain } (\varepsilon) = \frac{\text{change in length } (\Delta L)}{\text{original length } (L_0)}$$

where: ε = strain (no unit)
ΔL = change in length (m)
L_0 = original length (m)

Strain has **no units** because it is a ratio of lengths.

Tip: You need to memorise the equations for stress and strain in order to answer numerical questions in the exam.

5.1 MATERIAL PROPERTIES

Worked example
An unstretched wire is 1.20 m long. It is stretched by a force until extends by 1.15 mm. Calculate the strain in the wire.

Answer
Use the equation: $\text{strain} = \dfrac{\text{change in length}}{\text{original length}}$

First ensure that both lengths are in the same units.
$\Delta L = 1.15 \text{ mm} = 1.15 \times 10^{-3}$ m
(since 1 m = 1000 mm)
$L_O = 1.20$ m

$\text{strain }(\varepsilon) = \dfrac{\Delta L}{L_O} = \dfrac{1.15 \times 10^{-3}}{1.20} = 9.58 \times 10^{-4}$

> **Tip:** Always show all steps in your working out. Remember there are no units for strain.

The Young modulus (E)

The Young modulus is a measure of the stiffness of a material. It indicates how much a material will stretch (i.e., how much strain it will undergo) as a result of a given amount of stress. It can be used to compare the stiffness of different materials. The Young modulus can be calculated using the equation:

Young modulus (E) $= \dfrac{\text{stress }(\sigma)}{\text{strain }(\varepsilon)}$

Since strain does not have units, the Young modulus has the same units as stress (N m^{-2}).

A material that is stiff and fairly resistant to stretching has a high Young modulus value. For example, iron has a Young modulus of 2.1×10^{11} N m^{-2} whereas rubber, which is not stiff, has a much lower Young modulus of 2.0×10^{7} N m^{-2}.

It is important to note that the Young modulus **only applies up to the limit of proportionality** of a material. The limit of proportionality is the point up to which load is directly proportional to the extension. We will consider this point in more detail in a later section. However this fact allows us to define the Young modulus as follows:

Within the limit of proportionality, the ratio between stress and strain in a material is the Young modulus.

Worked example
A wire of length 2.0 m and diameter 0.40 mm is hung from the ceiling. Find the extension caused in the wire when a weight of 100 N is hung on it. The Young modulus (E) for the wire is 2.0×10^{11} N m^{-2}.

Answer
First write down the known data in the question:

$F = 100$ N

$L = 2.0$ m

$d = 0.40 \text{ mm} = \dfrac{0.40}{1000} = 4.0 \times 10^{-4}$ m

$E = 2.0 \times 10^{11}$ N m^{-2}

> **Tip:** The length and diameter must both be stated in metres.

The cross section area of the wire can first be calculated using:

$A = \dfrac{\pi d^2}{4} = \dfrac{\pi (4.0 \times 10^{-4})^2}{4} = 1.26 \times 10^{-7}$ m^2

Then calculate the stress using:

$\sigma = \dfrac{F}{A} = \dfrac{100}{1.26 \times 10^{-7}} = 8.0 \times 10^{8}$ N m^{-2}

Then use the equation:

$E = \dfrac{\sigma}{\varepsilon}$

$2.0 \times 10^{11} = \dfrac{8.0 \times 10^{8}}{\varepsilon}$

giving: $\varepsilon = \dfrac{8.0 \times 10^{8}}{2.0 \times 10^{11}} = 4.0 \times 10^{-3}$

Finally, to calculate the extension, ΔL, use the equation:

$\varepsilon = \dfrac{\Delta L}{L_O}$

$4.0 \times 10^{-3} = \dfrac{\Delta L}{2.0}$

giving: $\Delta L = 4.0 \times 10^{-3} \times 2.0 = 8.0 \times 10^{-3}$ m

> **Tip:** You need to practice answering questions like this. You must learn the equations for stress, strain and Young modulus well.

The Young modulus can also be calculated from a graph of stress against strain for a particular material. The gradient of such a graph is $\frac{stress}{strain}$ and is therefore equal to the Young modulus of that material. In the graph below, we can see that material X has a higher value of Young modulus than material Y because it has a steeper gradient. This means that material X is stiffer than material Y.

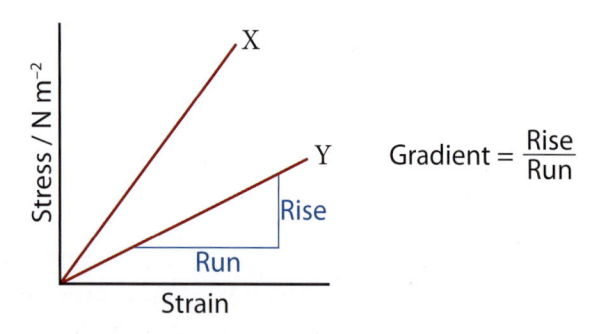

The gradient of a stress-strain graph gives the Young modulus

Experiment to determine stress, strain and the Young modulus for the material of a metal wire

This experiment involves loading a metal wire with weights and measuring the extension. Fixed weights can be used, or a newton meter can be used to check the weight of the load. The wire will be under tension, so safety goggles should be worn in case the wire breaks. The masses used are not very heavy but, nevertheless, care must be taken when adding and removing them.

> **Tip:** Check that there are no kinks in the wire before starting, otherwise the extension will be due to the kinks straightening out.

Method
- Hang a wire from the ceiling with a small (5 N) load attached to keep it taut. This is the reference wire.
- Attach to the ceiling another wire of the same material, cross section area and length. Both wires should be long (at least 2 m) so that the extension of the test wire will be large enough to measure – it will be a very small value. A vernier arrangement can be used, as shown in the diagram.
- Use a metre stick to measure and record the initial length (L_O) of the test wire in mm. The measurement should be taken from the point of suspension to the arrow on the Vernier scale.
- Using a micrometre screw gauge, measure the diameter, d, of the wire at several places. Calculate the average diameter and the cross section area of the wire using the equation: cross section area = $\frac{\pi d^2}{4}$.
- Increase the load, in steps of 10 N, measuring the extension from the vernier scale (in mm) each time.
- Calculate the stress ($\frac{F}{A}$) and strain ($\frac{\Delta L}{L_O}$) for each load.
- Plot a graph of stress (y-axis) against strain (x-axis). The gradient of this straight-line graph will be the Young modulus.

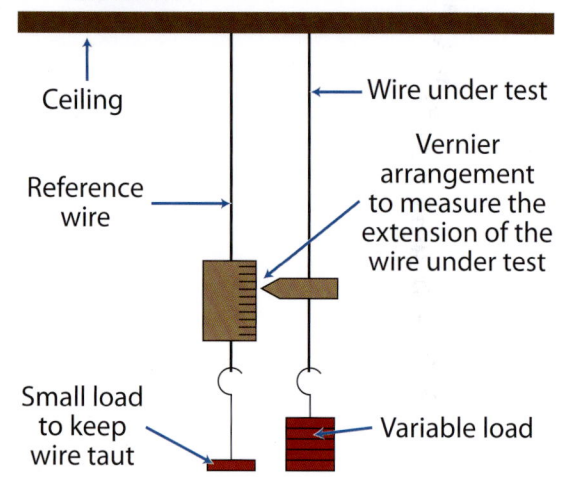

Alternative method
- Clamp a wire horizontally along a desk passing over a pulley to hang vertically, as shown in the diagram opposite.
- Use a metre stick to measure and record the initial length (L_O) of the test wire in mm, up to a reference mark.
- Measure the diameter of the wire as described above.
- Attach different loads in steps of 10 N and measure the extension using a mm scale.
- Calculate stress and strain for each load and plot a graph of stress against strain.
- This method is often used with a copper wire as steel stretches very little horizontally.

5.1 MATERIAL PROPERTIES

Diagram: Experimental setup showing wire under test attached to a marker, running over a pulley clamped to bench, with a variable load hanging. A metre stick is used with the marker on wire to help measure extension.

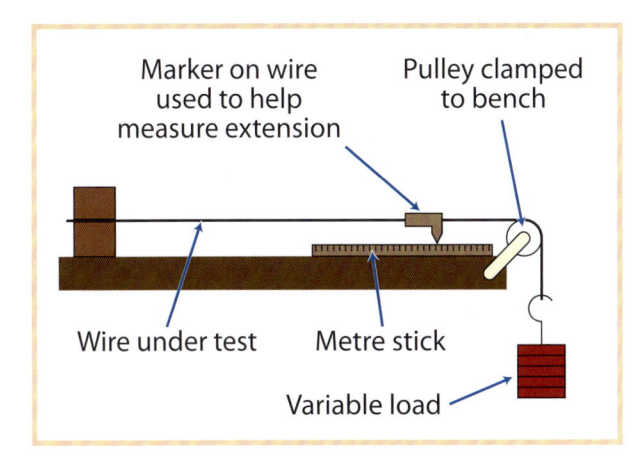

Elastic and plastic behaviour

If the experiment to determine stress, strain and the Young modulus is repeated for increasing loads on a wire, up to the point of fracture, a graph similar to that shown below is obtained.

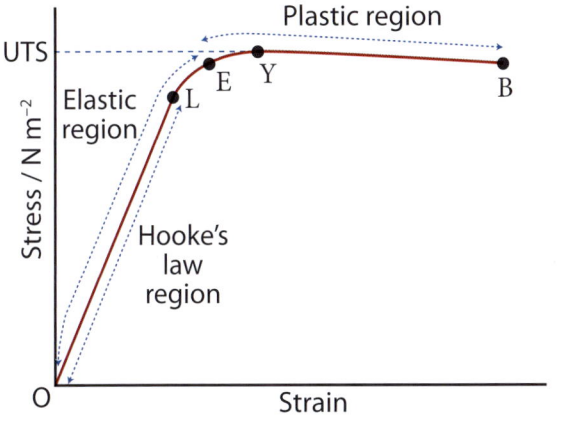

Stress-strain graph for a typical material, illustrating elastic and plastic behaviour. The graph shows Stress / N m^{-2} against Strain, with an Elastic region (Hooke's law region from O to L), then points L, E, Y and UTS marked, and a Plastic region extending to breaking point B.

Between point O and point L, this material is showing **elastic** behaviour. **A material is showing elastic behaviour when it returns to its original dimensions following tension or compression.** Elastic materials obey Hooke's law, which states that the extension is proportional to the force applied (i.e. stress is proportional to strain) and the graph is a straight line. The material obeys Hooke's law between points O and L.

> **Tip:** When stretching a material, the **limit of proportionality** is the point beyond which Hooke's law is no longer true.

Point L is the **limit of proportionality**. Between points L and E the graph is no longer a straight line but bends. However, even though the material has stopped obeying Hooke's law in this region, it would still return to original shape if the stress was removed. It is therefore still displaying elastic behaviour.

Point E is called the **elastic limit**. **The elastic limit is the maximum load a specimen can experience and still return to its original length when the deforming force is removed.** If the material is stressed beyond its elastic limit, it starts to undergo permanent deformation. This is called **plastic behaviour**. **A material is showing plastic behaviour when it undergoes permanent deformation when in a state of tension or compression.** It can no longer return to its original shape and size even when the deforming force is removed.

Point Y is the **yield strength**. **Yield strength is that stress at which elastic deformation ends and plastic deformation begins.** At this point, the structure of the material starts to break down and small increases in stress cause a massive increase in extension (strain).

> **Tip:** The **yield strength** marks the point where there is a large permanent change in length with no extra load.

As the stress is increased, the material continues to deform until it eventually breaks or fractures at point B. This is called the **breaking point** (or fracture point). The maximum stress that a material will withstand before breaking is called the **ultimate tensile strength** (UTS). Ultimate tensile strength is the maximum stress that a material can withstand while being stretched or pulled before breaking.

> **Tip:** You should be able to determine the UTS value from a stress-strain graph: it is the highest value that the stress reaches.

> **Tip:** An experiment to determine the Young modulus can be continued until the wire breaks, and a graph plotted. This will show the elastic and plastic region.

Drawing conclusions from stress-strain graphs

Different materials have different stress-strain graphs, and such graphs can be used to draw conclusions about materials.

Brittle materials

Brittle materials, such as glass or cast iron, are very stiff. These materials will behave elastically and obey Hooke's law when a stress is applied to them. However when the load is increased they will fracture with no warning and without displaying plastic deformation. A stress-strain graph for a brittle material is shown below.

Ductile materials

Ductility is a measure of the ability of a material to be drawn into a wire. Most metals are ductile whereas ceramics are not. A ductile material such as copper can be easily and permanently stretched. The graph below shows that a ductile material initially behaves elastically and obeys Hooke's law. However there is then a large plastic region within which the material will continue to stretch. Even if the stress is reduced the material will be permanently stretched. It eventually breaks.

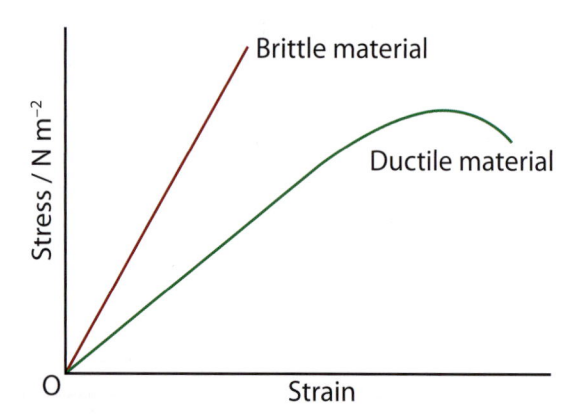

Stress-strain graphs for a brittle and ductile material

> **Tip:** Notice that the ductile material in the graph is the weaker of the two as it has the lower ultimate tensile strength (UTS).

> **Tip:** You can tell that the Young modulus for the brittle material is the greater of the two, because the gradient is greater.

Polymers

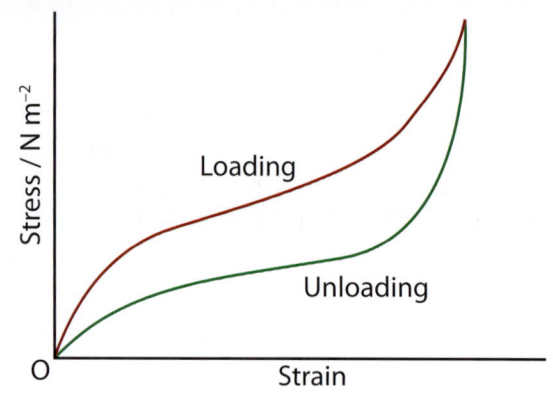

Stress-strain graph for a polymer

A polymer, such as rubber, has its molecules arranged in long chains that are initially coiled and tangled. When a stress is applied, the chains straighten out, resulting in a large strain. As a result, polymers can undergo much larger strains for a small stress than other materials.

The graph above shows a stress-strain graph for a typical polymer. Polymeric materials have no elastic (linear) region on the graph. The material will not go back to its original length after bring strained. When the load is first applied, the material is quite stiff. As the stress is increased, only a small strain is observed and the gradient of the graph is high, because the polymer chains are beginning to uncoil. As the stress is increased, however, the chains become straighter and the stiffness decreases. At this point, small increases in stress will produce a large strain, and the gradient of the graph decreases. Finally, the chains become completely uncoiled and the stiffness increases once again, approaching the stiffness of the chains themselves.

The stress-strain curve for a polymer is different when unloading than when loading. This is known as **hysteresis**, and the two curves make a hysteresis loop. The area under a stress-strain curve is equal to the energy per unit volume stored by the material on loading or released on unloading. It shows that rubber is not a very good material for storing energy. In one loading and unloading cycle, the energy represented by the area bound by the hysteresis loop is lost, usually as heat.

Creep and fatigue strength

Creep and fatigue are types of deformation that eventually result in the failure of materials. It is vital for engineers to have an understanding of these concepts when choosing materials for machinery or structures.

5.1 MATERIAL PROPERTIES

Creep

Creep is the continuous slow deformation (change in shape) that occurs when a material is under **constant** stress over time.

When a material is subjected to a constant load for a long time, creep can cause plastic deformation even below the yield point. The effect of creep is greater at higher temperatures, but some metals, such as lead and tin, show creep even at room temperature. For example, lead used in roofing gradually becomes deformed under its own weight due to creep. Similarly, many electrical cables are taut when first installed but after some time they sag due to creep. Sometimes the effect of creep can be so large that it affects function. For example, creep of a turbine blade in a jet engine will cause the blade to lengthen, and it could eventually come into contact with the casing and fail.

Fatigue

Fatigue is the deformation that occurs when a material is repeatedly being stressed and having the stress removed.

It is difficult to break a metal wire by stretching it, but if the wire is bent and unbent repeatedly, it breaks easily. This is known as cyclic loading. Many rotating machine parts are subjected to repeated cycles of stress caused by rotation or vibration (e.g. the components of a car) and can fail due to fatigue.

Fatigue failure starts with a small crack appearing due to repeated working. Once a crack has formed, stress builds up and the crack enlarges until the material eventually fractures. When choosing materials for a purpose, it is important to look at the material's **fatigue strength**. The fatigue strength is the stress that will produce failure within a set number of cycles.

> **Tip:** Make sure you understand the difference between creep and fatigue. Creep occurs slowly over time. Fatigue is caused by repeated loading and unloading.

Questions

1. Calculate the density of a 500 g rectangular block with a length of 8.1 cm, width of 6.0 cm, and height of 5.0 cm. **[2 marks]**

2. A glass block has dimensions 0.36 m × 0.55 m × 0.0025 m. It has mass 1.30 kg. Calculate the density of the block in kg m^{-3} and in g m^{-3}. **[3 marks]**

3. A block of copper has volume of 0.00050 m^3. The density of copper is 9.0×10^3 kg m^{-3}. Calculate the mass of the block. **[2 marks]**

4. Calculate the mass of a cement pillar that is 1.5 m wide, 2.0 m deep and 3.0 m high. The density of concrete is 2400 kg m^{-3}. **[2 marks]**

5. A solution is made up by adding a mass of sodium chloride to 250 cm^3 of water to form a sodium chloride solution of density 1.07 g cm^{-3}. The density of pure water is 1.00 g cm^{-3}. Calculate the mass of sodium chloride present in the sodium chloride solution, assuming that the volume of water stays at 250 cm^3 when salt is added. **[4 marks]**

6. Define the following terms:
   (a) thermal conductivity [1]
   (b) electrical conductivity [1]
   (c) chemical resistance [1] **[3 marks]**

7. Name a material that has:
   (a) a high thermal conductivity [1]
   (b) a low thermal conductivity [1] **[2 marks]**

8. To test for chemical resistance material A and material B were placed into separate beakers of hydrochloric acid. Material A fizzed and decreased in size. Material B darkened in colour. Deduce from the experimental results which material is more chemically resistant. Explain your answer. **[2 marks]**

9. What is the electrical conductivity of a nichrome wire of length 0.25 m, cross section area 6.0×10^{-8} m^2 and resistance 4.2 Ω? **[3 marks]**

10. State the name of an instrument used to measure the diameter of a wire. **[1 mark]**

11. (a) State the equation used to calculate the cross section area of a wire. [1]
    (b) What is the effect on the cross section area of the wire if the diameter of the wire is doubled? [1] **[2 marks]**

12. (a) Name and describe the type of material that is used to indent the test material in the Vickers test. [3]
    (b) State the size of the force load used in the Vickers test and the length of time it is applied for. [2]
    (c) State the units of hardness used in the Vickers test. [1] **[6 marks]**

13. When determining the Young modulus for the material of a wire experimentally, a stress is applied to the wire and a strain produced.
    (a) Define the terms stress, strain and Young modulus. [3]
    (b) When carrying out this experiment, a series of masses are hung on a wire and measurements recorded. List the measurements you would make and state how and with what equipment they would be taken. [4]
    (c) Explain why a long wire is most suitable for this experiment. [1] **[8 marks]**

14. An elastic cord of unstretched length 160 mm has a cross section area of 0.64 mm². It is stretched to a length of 190 mm. The Young modulus for the cord is 2.0×10^7 N m^{-2}. Calculate the force (tension) in the cord at this extension. **[4 marks]**

15. A vertical steel piano wire of length 1.5 m and cross section area of 1.3×10^{-6} m² supports a load of 80 N. Given that the Young modulus for steel is 2.0×10^{11} N m^{-2}, calculate the extension in the wire produced by this load. **[5 marks]**

16. Some stress and strain graphs for different wires are shown below.
    (a) In figure 1, state what is represented by each of points A, B, C and D. [4]
    (b) State which wire in figure 2, E or F, has a greater Young modulus, and explain how you can determine this. [2]
    (c) State which wire in figure 3, G or H, is more brittle, and explain how you can determine this. [2] **[8 marks]**

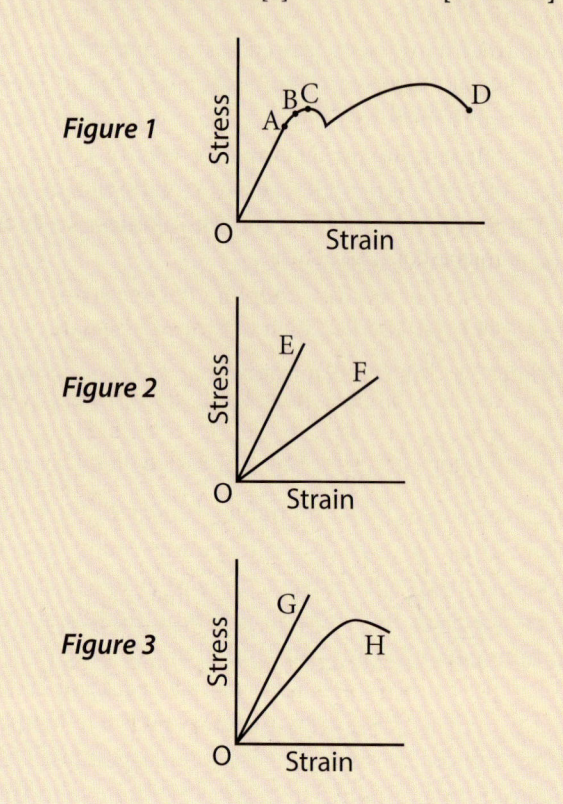

Figure 1

Figure 2

Figure 3

5.2–5.3 CATEGORISING MATERIALS AND MICROSCOPIC STRUCTURE

Students should be able to:

5.2.1 investigate a range of general materials that can be grouped into distinct categories, and be aware of metals, ceramics, glasses, polymers and composites;

5.2.2 give examples of materials in each of the categories investigated and justify their use in a range of situations;

5.3.1 label a diagram of a Bohr model atom (knowledge of sub-orbitals is not required);

5.3.2 describe how the properties of metals relate to microscopic structure;

5.3.3 describe how the properties of crystalline, amorphous and polymeric materials relate to microscopic structure;

5.3.4 demonstrate an understanding that thermosets are polymers that strengthen while being heated and cannot be remoulded after they are initially formed because they have cross-links between the polymer chains;

5.3.5 demonstrate an understanding that thermoplastics are polymers that soften when heated and then harden and strengthen on cooling, and that they can be remoulded after they are initially formed because they have no cross-links between the polymer chains;

5.3.6 explain typical uses of thermosetting and thermoplastics;

5.3.7 describe how the properties of composite materials relate to microscopic structure; and

5.3.8 investigate the crystal structure of a range of materials using a polarising light microscope.

The Bohr model of an atom

Atoms are the building blocks of all materials. The **Bohr model** describes the atom as a small, positively charged nucleus containing positively charged protons and neutral neutrons, surrounded by negatively charged electrons that move in shells.

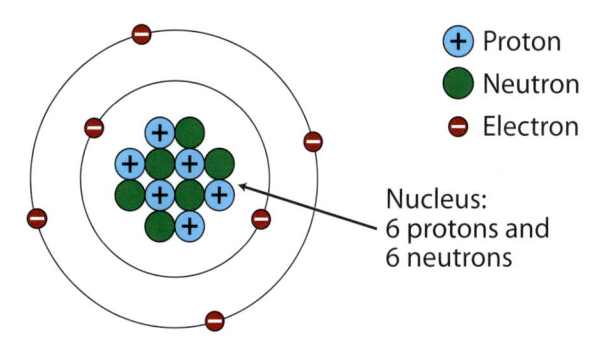

The Bohr model, showing the structure of a carbon atom

Tip: Atoms have a neutral charge overall because they have an equal number of protons and electrons.

Each atom has an **atomic number**, which gives the number of protons in the atom. Because atoms have a neutral charge, the atomic number also equals the number of electrons in the atom. Each atom also has a **mass number** that gives the total number of protons and neutrons. This can be summarised as follows:

Number of protons
= number of electrons = atomic number

Number of neutrons
= mass number − atomic number

These numbers are often written in the form $^A_B X$ where X is the symbol for the element, A is the mass number and B is the atomic number.

Worked example
How many protons, neutrons and electrons are in an atom of sodium $^{23}_{11}Na$.

Answer
Number of protons = number of electrons
= atomic number
= 11
Number of neutrons
= mass number − atomic number
= 23 − 11
= 12
So the atom contains 11 protons, 11 electrons and 12 neutrons.

In an atom, electrons are arranged in **shells** or **energy levels**. Electrons occupy the lowest energy levels first. The first shell, which is closest to the nucleus and can hold up to two electrons, is filled first. The second shell, which can hold up to eight electrons, is filled next. The third shell can also hold up to eight electrons.

> **Worked example**
> Draw and write the electronic arrangement (electronic configuration) of phosphorus, which has atomic number 15.
>
> **Answer**
> Number of electrons = atomic number = 15.
> The first shell holds 2 electrons, this leaves 13 electrons.
> The second shell holds 8 electrons, this leaves 5 electrons.
> The third shell has 5 electrons. 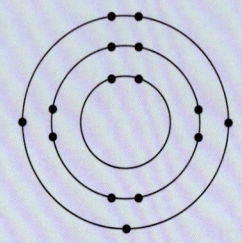
>
> This is written as: 2,8,5.

shown in the diagram. The metal ions are fixed in a regular position, but they do vibrate. The metallic bond is the attraction between the positive ions and the delocalised electrons. It is a strong attraction.

Tip: A positive **ion** is formed when an atom loses electrons. The lost electrons become **delocalised**. Delocalised electrons are electrons that do not have fixed positions but move freely.

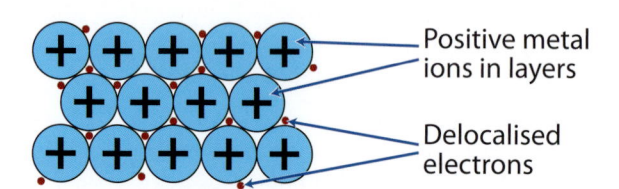

The structure of a metal

Tip: Make sure you are able to draw and label this diagram.

Understanding this structure allows us to explain the properties of metals:
- Metals are **good conductors of electricity** because the delocalised electrons can move and carry charge.
- Metals are **good conductors of heat** because the delocalised electrons can move and carry heat energy. When a metal is heated, the delocalised electrons gain heat energy, which causes them to move more rapidly and randomly. The metal ions in the lattice also vibrate more when a metal is heated. The delocalised electrons collide with vibrating metal ions in the lattice. These collisions increase the kinetic energy of the lattice ions and so they in turn can pass on or conduct the energy more quickly. This process results in an increase in temperature along the metal away from the point of heating.
- Metals have **high melting points** because the metallic bonds (the attraction between the positive ions and delocalised electrons) are strong and it takes substantial energy to break them. The metal will turn into a liquid only when these bonds are broken.
- Metals are **malleable** and **ductile** because the layers of ions can slide over each other. Despite this sliding, the delocalised electrons still attract the ions and therefore hold the structure together – the metallic bonding is not disrupted.

Categorising Materials

Materials can be grouped into categories depending on their **structure**. Structure describes how the atoms or ions are arranged in space. By understanding the structure of materials in each category at a microscopic level, it is possible to explain their properties.

In this section we will look at the following categories and their structure:
- metals
- ceramics
- glasses
- polymers
- composites

Metals

The structure of a metal is a giant lattice of **positive ions** arranged in regular layers, with **delocalised** electrons free to move throughout the structure, as

- Metals have a **crystalline** structure. A crystalline structure is a **regular or ordered arrangement of particles**. If a metal is examined under a polarising light microscope, tiny crystals can be seen. They seldom form into one giant crystal.

Ceramics

Ceramics are earthenware, porcelain or china materials produced by moulding and firing in a hot kiln. The atoms in ceramics are joined by **strong covalent (or sometimes ionic) bonds**, which makes them harder and more rigid than metals. They are chemically resistant and tend to be good thermal and electrical insulators as the ions can't move and carry charge. Ceramics are brittle, as there are no layers to slide over each other, but are hard and strong when compressed. Ceramic bricks are used in construction, ceramic tiles are used in kitchens, and new ceramics made from zinc oxide are used in semiconductors and resistors.

Glasses

Glasses are amorphous structures. An **amorphous** structure is one which has **no regular arrangement of particles**, the opposite of a crystalline structure. Glasses are made in a similar way to ceramics and have the same properties (i.e. glasses are good thermal and electrical insulators, are brittle, and are hard and strong when compressed). Glasses are often transparent and for this reason they are commonly used for drinking vessels, windows and lenses.

Polymers

A polymer is a large molecule made of many repeated units called monomers joined in a long chain molecule as shown in the diagram. Polymers may be classified as either **thermoset** (short for 'thermosetting plastic') or **thermoplastic**. The properties of thermosets and thermoplastics are summarised in the table on the next page.

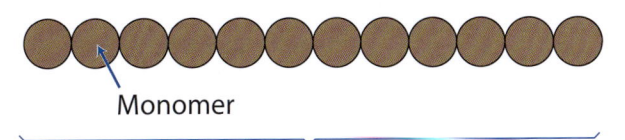

A representation of a polymer

The chains that make up a polymer can be arranged in different ways. Some polymers, such as high density poly(ethene), have straight chains that pack together closely so they are hard and rigid. Other polymers, such as low density poly(ethene), have branched chains that do not fit together as closely and as a result they are more flexible.

Plasticisers are chemical substances that can be added to a polymer like PVC to hold the chains apart and therefore make it softer and more flexible. For this reason, plasticised PVC is used in electrical wire insulation, clothing and wellington boots. Unplasticised PVC is harder and more rigid and is therefore suitable for applications such as window frames and drainpipes.

> **Tip:** You may be asked to state properties that make a polymer suitable for a particular use. For example, plasticised poly(vinylchloride) is used in drainpipes and windows because it is chemically resistant, hard-wearing, light, rigid and waterproof.

> **Tip:** When explaining properties related to uses, do not refer to cost. Cost is not a property of the material.

Polymers often have **both crystalline and amorphous** regions. Such materials may be referred to as **semi-crystalline** polymers. In the crystalline areas, the chains are regularly arranged but in the amorphous regions they are tangled and disordered, as shown in the diagram. Highly ordered chains make the material strong but brittle, so the presence of amorphous regions allows the polymer to bend without breaking.

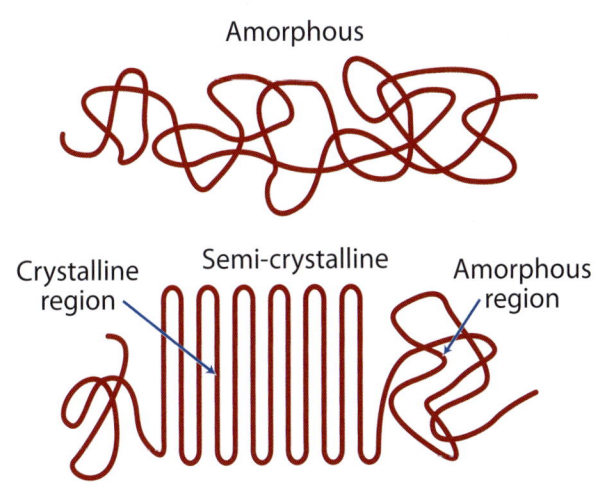

The structure of chains in amorphous and semi-crystalline polymers

	Thermosets	Thermoplastics
Molecular structure	There are **strong crosslinks** (covalent bonds) between the polymer chains. These bonds are difficult to break even when heated.	There are **no crosslinks** between the polymer chains, just weak intermolecular forces. These forces are easily broken on heating.
Definition	Thermosets are polymers that strengthen while being heated and cannot be remoulded after they are initially formed because of the strong crosslinks between the polymer chains. They do not melt.	Thermoplastics are polymers that soften when heated and then harden and strengthen on cooling. They can be remoulded after they are initially formed because they have no crosslinks between the polymer chains.
Diagram	Crosslinks	Chains
General properties	Rigid and high strength, heat resistant, chemically resistant, lightweight.	Not stiff, waterproof, only used at temperatures below 125°C, chemically resistant, lightweight.
Examples	**melamine** – used in laminate kitchen worktops, toilet seats, picnic cups and plates. **bakelite** – used in saucepan handles and light socket fittings, radio casings, doorknobs. **urea formaldehyde** – used in electrical fittings, control knobs, adhesives.	**low density poly(ethene) (LDPE)** – used in cling film, carrier bags, bottles. **high density poly(ethene) (HDPE)** – used in water pipes and garden furniture. **acrylic** – used in baths and windows. **unplasticised poly(vinylchloride) (uPVC)** – used in drain pipes, window frames. **plasticised poly(vinylchloride) (PVC)** – used in wellington boots, clothes, electric wire insulation.

Composites

A composite is created by combining different materials to create one that has better, more useful properties than any of its components. Some composites are easy to make. Others are difficult to fabricate and are therefore expensive.

Aluminium alloys are lightweight and are traditionally used in situations where weight is important. However, **carbon fibre reinforced plastic** is a composite that is even less dense, so it is often used in modern aircraft. The advantage of using this material is that the plane is lighter and needs less fuel.

Steel reinforced concrete is a composite made from a mesh of steel cables set in concrete. Concrete is strong if compressed but weak when stretched. However, the steel makes the material strong when stretched so the composite combines the properties of both materials to create a material with more suitable properties. Steel reinforced concrete is used in the construction of buildings and bridges.

There are many other examples of composites. **Bone** and **wood** are both natural composites. Bone is made from a hard, brittle material called hydroxyapatite (which is mainly calcium phosphate) and a soft, flexible material called collagen (which is a protein). On its own, collagen would be useless in a skeleton, but when combined with hydroxyapatite it gives bone the properties needed to support the body. Wood is made from long cellulose fibres held together by an even weaker substance called lignin. Cellulose is also found in cotton, but without the lignin to bind it together, it is much weaker. Despite both lignin and cellulose being weak substances, together they form a much stronger material.

Medium density fibreboard (MDF) is a composite made from wood fibres and glue. **Glass reinforced plastic** is a composite made of a woven mat of glass fibre soaked in a thermosetting plastic resin; it is strong and very light and used in boats and car bodies.

Using a polarising light microscope

A polarising light microscope can be used to look at the **crystal structure** of a range of materials. A regular light microscope uses unpolarised white light. In **unpolarised** light waves, the **vibrations occur in every possible plane** perpendicular to the direction of the light propagation. However, a polarising light microsope uses **polarised** light. In polarised light, the **vibrations occur in only one plane** perpendicular to the direction of the light propagation. The use of polarised light improves contrast, and hence image quality, when examining **aniosotropic** materials. An anisotropic material is one that has a physical property that has a different value when measured in different directions. Wood is an example of an anisotopic material because is stronger along the grain than across it. Polarised light microscopy gives information about the molecular structure of a material.

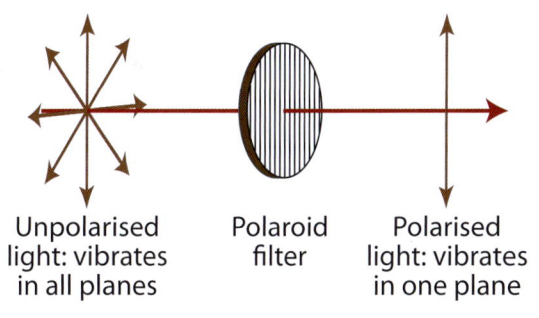

Unpolarised light: vibrates in all planes — Polaroid filter — Polarised light: vibrates in one plane

Passing unpolarised light through a polaroid filter produces polarised light

A standard light microscope can be converted into a polarising light microscope by adding two polaroid filters called a **polariser** and an **analyser.** The **polariser** is positioned in the light path beneath the material under the microscope stage and can be rotated through 360°. It helps to polarise the light that falls on the material. The **analyser** is placed above the microscope's objective lens. It combines the different rays emerging from the specimen to generate the final image. When both filters are initially aligned in the light path, they are at right angles to each other. When rotated by different amounts, light is able to pass through the filters at different angles, allowing the viewer to see different aspects of the specimen. Rotating the polariser will cause different parts to black out (extinction) at different times.

When an anisotropic material, such as wood, is brought into focus and rotated through 360° in the microscope it will sequentially appear bright and dark (extinct), depending upon the rotation position. When the material's long axis is oriented at a 45° angle to the polariser axis, the maximum degree of brightness will be achieved. The greatest degree of extinction will be observed when the two axes coincide. During rotation over a range of 360°, the material's visibility will oscillate between bright and dark four times, in 90° increments.

Questions

1. (a) In the Bohr model of the atom:
   (i) name the particles found in the nucleus [1]
   (ii) name the negative particles in the atom and state where they are found [1]
   (iii) name the positive particles in the atom and state where they are found. [1]
   (b) With reference to the Bohr model, explain why atoms have no charge. [1] **[4 marks]**

2. Explain why metals are good conductors of electricity. **[2 marks]**

3. Explain why metals are malleable. **[2 marks]**

4. Explain whether metals are crystalline or amorphous. **[1 mark]**

5. Explain what is meant by the term 'polymer'. **[2 marks]**

6. Explain the difference between a thermopolymer and a thermoset in terms of their structure. **[4 marks]**

7. The diagrams below show the structure of two plastics.

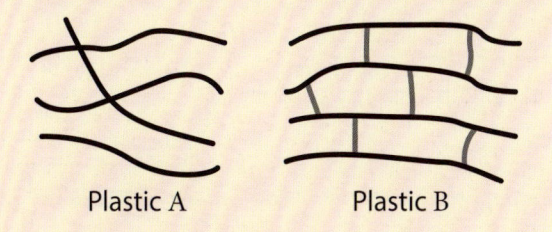

   Plastic A   Plastic B

   (a) Explain why plastic A can be easily stretched. [2]
   (b) Explain why plastic B has a high melting point. [2] **[4 marks]**

8. What is a composite material? **[2 marks]**

5.4–5.5 ALLOYS, METAL WORKING AND BIOMATERIALS

Students should be able to

5.4.1 describe what an alloy is;

5.4.2 investigate practically and compare the physical properties of bronze, brass and stainless steel;

5.4.3 give examples of alloys, their constituent materials and common uses, including steel, stainless steel, invar, bronze, brass and nichrome;

5.4.4 demonstrate an understanding that annealing is a heat treatment of metals to make them softer, easier to work and easier to cut;

5.4.5 describe annealing as the heating of a metal to a temperature above its recrystallization temperature and then letting it cool slowly;

5.4.6 analyse data relating to the constituent make-up of alloys and resulting properties to arrive at a decision about the suitability of a particular alloy for a given task;

5.5.1 recall that a biomaterial is one that is inserted into the body as part of a medical device;

5.5.2 recall that a bioinert material is one that does not release toxins, is not rejected by the body and does not react with biological tissue;

5.5.3 recall that a bioactive material is one that does react with adjacent biological tissues in the body; and

5.5.4 recall that biotolerant materials are those that are not rejected when implanted into the living tissue but are surrounded by a fibrous layer in the form of a capsule and that there are negligible toxins released.

Alloys

An alloy is a mixture of two or more elements, of which at least one is a metal, and where the resulting mixture has metallic properties.

Alloys often have properties that are different to the metals they contain. This makes them more useful than the pure metals alone. For example, alloys are often harder than the pure metals.

The CCEA specification requires you have knowledge of six alloys in particular. The table below gives their names, their constituent materials, physical properties and some common uses.

Alloy	Constituent materials	Physical properties	Common uses
steel	iron (80–98%), carbon (0.2–2%), plus small amounts of other metals such as chromium, manganese and vanadium.	Strong, hard, rusts.	Car bodies, bridges, ships.
stainless steel	iron (50%+), chromium (10–30%), plus smaller amounts of carbon, nickel and manganese.	Shiny, strong and resists rusting. Less brittle than steel.	Medical tools, cutlery, storage tanks for food products, machine parts.
invar	iron (64%), nickel (36%).	Low thermal expansion.	Thermostats, clock and watch mechanisms.
bronze	copper (90%), tin (5–10%), plus manganese, phosphorus, aluminium or silicon.	Very ductile, hard, strong, shiny, resistant to corrosion, conducts electricity (better conductor of electricity than steel).	Statues, ships' propellers, bells and cymbals.
brass	copper (70%), zinc (30%).	Hard, shiny, resistant to corrosion, very malleable, easier to cast than steel.	Door locks and bolts, musical instruments.
nichrome	nickel (80%), chromium (20%).	Very strong, resistant to corrosion.	Firework ignition devices, flame test wires, heating elements in electrical appliances.

5.4–5.5 ALLOYS, METAL WORKING AND BIOMATERIALS

Tip: Note that most metals corrode, but only iron (and some iron alloys) rust. Rust is hydrated iron(III) oxide. Rusting is a type of corrosion, a chemical reaction that causes the metal to be destroyed.

Tip: You need to learn the constituent materials and common uses of **all** the alloys in the table, but the CCEA specification only requires you to know the **physical properties** of bronze, brass and stainless steel.

It is possible to practically investigate the properties of alloys. For example, bronze, brass and stainless steel can be compared for hardness using the Vickers method. The alloys can also be investigated for thermal and electrical conductivity and for melting point.

Tip: In an exam question, you might be given data about the properties of different alloys, and be asked to determine which alloy is most suitable for a particular use.

Worked example
The table below gives information about some different alloys: A, B, C and D.

Alloy	Constituent elements	Properties
A	Bismuth, cadmium, lead and tin.	Melts at 70°C.
B	Carbon, iron and tungsten.	Unaffected at high temperatures. High strength.
C	Copper and zinc.	Golden colour, does not tarnish or corrode.
D	Aluminium and lithium.	Low density, high strength.

Which alloy would be most suitable for use in
(a) making jewellery?
(b) making aircraft bodywork?
(c) making a drill for bricks and stone?

Answer
(a) C is best for jewellery due to its attractive golden colour and the fact that it does not corrode or tarnish.
(b) D is best for aircraft manufacture, as it is light yet strong.
(c) B is best for drills, as it is strong and is not affected by the high temperatures that may occur when the drill is rotating into the brick.

Annealing

Annealing is a heat treatment of metals to make them softer, easier to work and easier to cut.

The annealing procedure involves heating the alloy or metal to a high temperature (above its recrystallization temperature) and keeping it at this temperature for some time. It is then allowed to cool, usually slowly, to below its recrystallization temperature.

Biomaterials

A biomaterial is a material that is inserted into the human body as part of a medical device. Biomaterials play an important role in modern medicine by restoring function or facilitating healing for people after injury or disease. Examples of medical devices made from biomaterials are stainless steel heart stents, titanium pacemakers, synthetic skin and metal hip or knee joints.

Biomaterials are classified into three distinct categories, based on the reaction of living tissue to the biomaterial:

- **Biotolerant materials** are those that are not rejected when implanted into living tissue but are surrounded by a fibrous layer in the form of a capsule and that release negligible toxins. Typical biotolerant materials are glass, silicone, most metals and synthetic polymers.

Tip: Rejection means that the body tries to attack or destroy the material added.

- **A bioinert material** is one that does not release toxins, is not rejected by the body and does not react with biological tissue in the body. They can usually be in direct contact

115

with bone. Typical bioinert implant materials include stainless steel, titanium and zirconium.

- **A bioactive material** is one that does react with adjacent biological tissues in the body. Such materials often form bonds with bone. An example of a bioactive material is bioglass, which enhances bone formation when used in implants in patients. Bioglass interacts with living tissue by taking part in ion transfer inside the body and forming a fibrous capsule around the implant.

> **Tip:** You need to learn the difference between these types of biomaterial.

Questions

1. Explain why brass is classified as an alloy. [2 marks]
2. Name two constituents of invar. [2 marks]
3. Compare the constituents of steel with stainless steel. [3 marks]
4. Name the two main elements present in bronze. [2 marks]
5. State two uses for brass. [2 marks]
6. State two uses for invar. [2 marks]
7. Describe the process of annealing. [3 marks]
8. State the purpose of annealing. [1 mark]
9. Name two devices that are made from biomaterials. [2 marks]
10. Explain the difference between a bioinert material and a bioactive material. [2 marks]
11. Tricalcium phosphate is used in dental implants and causes direct chemical bonding between bone and the dental implant. Explain whether calcium phosphate ceramic is bioinert or bioactive. [1 mark]
12. Stainless steel is used in bone screws. State two of the properties that this alloy has that make it suitable for this use. [2 marks]
13. Name a material suitable for a hip joint replacement. [1 mark]
14. Define the term 'biomaterial'. [1 mark]

5.6, 5.7, 5.9 SMART MATERIALS, NANOMATERIALS AND INDUSTRIAL CONSIDERATIONS

Students should be able to:

5.6.1 define a smart material and investigate the properties of a range of smart materials;

5.6.2 briefly outline the defining features of shape-memory alloys, piezoelectric materials, quantum-tunneling composites, thermochromatic materials, photochromic materials and electroluminescent materials;

5.6.3 apply knowledge of smart material features to specific situations;

5.7.1 describe the structure of graphite, graphene and a carbon nanotube;

5.7.2 demonstrate an understanding of the physical properties of carbon nanotubes;

5.7.3 evaluate the potential uses for carbon nanotubes in health care (for example nitric oxide sensors, drug loading capacity, selective cancer cell destruction, bio-stress sensors, glucose detection biosensors and scaffolding for tissue regeneration);

5.7.4 evaluate the benefits and risks of nanotechnology to society; and

5.9.1 evaluate the external factors that influence the choice of material for a particular situation – price, environmental considerations, quality required, demand and regulations.

Smart materials

Smart materials have physical properties that change in response to an external condition, such as temperature, light, pressure or electricity. The change in the smart material is reversible and can be repeated many times. There are many different types of smart material, six of which are discussed in this section.

Thermochromatic materials

Thermochromatic materials **change colour** in response to a **change in temperature**. In medicine, these materials can be used in the manufacture of forehead thermometers. Test strips on the side of batteries are also made from thermochromatic materials (in this case the heat comes from a resistor under the thermochromatic film). In the food industry, thermochromatic inks can be used to indicate when a packaged food has reached the correct temperature in an oven.

Photochromic materials

Photochromic materials **change colour** reversibly in response to a **change in light**. They are usually colourless in a dark place, but when exposed to sunlight or ultraviolet radiation, the molecular structure of the material changes and they exhibit colour. When the relevant light source is removed the colour disappears again. Photochromic materials are used in the lenses of some sunglasses so that they become darker or lighter depending on the light conditions. Photochromic windows change their transparency in response to the amount of light, reducing glare and helping to prevent cooling systems in buildings from overloading in very sunny weather.

Electroluminescent materials

Electroluminescent materials **give out light** when an electric **current** is applied to them. They have a low power consumption, have a long life and can be shaped to be very flat. They are used in night lights, watch illumination systems, decorative luminescent clothing and, more recently, in computer monitors and billboards.

Shape-memory alloys (SMA)

A shape-memory alloy is an alloy that, when deformed, returns to its original shape when heated. This is a useful property in situations where a response to a change in temperature is needed, for example in controllers for hot water valves in showers and to activate sprinklers in fire alarm systems.

Other examples include spectacle frames, which are often made of a shape memory alloy called nitinol. The nitinol frames can be bent, but they can be returned to their original shape by heating. In medicine, doctors can use smart alloys to hold bones in place while they heal. They cool the alloy and then wrap it around the broken bone. When it heats up again, it returns to its original shape, pulling the bones together and holding them for healing. The same process can be used to insert stents (a tube inserted into a damaged blood vessel to prevent it from collapsing or bursting). Cold nitinol stents can be compressed in order to be inserted into a blood vessel. They then expand to the correct diameter at body temperature, keeping the blood vessel open. Shape-memory alloy wires are used in dental braces. The brace wire is first moulded to follow the shape of the teeth. After it is placed in the mouth it heats up and tries to reform into a straighter shape, exerting a constant force on the teeth and drawing them into the correct position. The disadvantages of smart alloys are their high cost and the risk of metal fatigue.

> **Tip:** Shape-memory alloy wires used in braces must be both chemically resistant and biotolerant.

Piezoelectric materials

A piezoelectric material **produces a voltage** when put under **stress** (e.g. when a mechanical force is used to bend or change their shape by squeezing). This process also works in reverse, so when a **voltage** is applied to a piezoelectric material it **changes shape**. The piezoelectric effect is found in nature – bone and quartz are both natural materials that have a piezoelectric effect.

Electronic cigarette lighters utilise the piezoelectric effect. Pressing the button causes a spring-loaded hammer to hit a piezoelectric material, producing an electric current that flows across a small spark gap to ignite the gas.

In sport, piezoelectric fibres can be embedded in tennis racquets with a computer chip placed in the handle. When the ball hits the racquet, the piezoelectric material is stressed and produces a voltage, which travels to the computer chip. The voltage is then boosted and sent back to the fibres in the racquet to reduce their vibration. This means the racquet transmits less shock vibration to the player.

Other devices that use piezoelectric materials are airbag sensors, keyless door entry systems, seat belt sensors and sensor mats.

Quantum-tunneling composites (QTCs)

Quantum-tunneling composites are flexible polymers that contain tiny metal particles. A QTC is normally an **insulator**, but if it is **squeezed**, it becomes a **conductor**. Without pressure, the conductive elements are too far apart to conduct electricity. However, when pressure is applied, they move closer and electrons can 'tunnel' through the insulator. QTCs are durable, inert materials and are unaffected by humidity.

Applications of QTCs include pressure sensors, motor speed controllers and, more recently, in touchscreens for smartphones, which eliminate the need for buttons. QTCs may also be used in touch switches in game controllers and computer mice, replacing conventional switches and sensors and giving increased sensitivity for greater control. Switches made from QTCs have the advantage that there are no mechanical parts, so they are durable and robust, and are ideal for applications which require spark-free operation (e.g. when working with fuel).

QTC switches are flexible, durable and washable and can therefore be incorporated into clothes (e.g. to allow the wearer to change music tracks or adjust the volume on their mobile phone, with switches attached to the phone via a connector in the inside pocket). Similar switches can be used in interactive dance mats to sense the movements of the user's feet. QTCs can also be used to make musical instruments. A keyboard using QTC switches for the keys is more flexible, durable and portable than a conventional keyboard.

Nanomaterials

Nanomaterials are composed of nanoparticles, which are between 1–100 nm (1 nm = 10^{-9} m) across. Particles of this size have a very high surface area to volume ratio and this means that the properties of nanomaterials are very different to that of the bulk material. New uses for nanomaterials are being researched and discovered daily.

Graphite, graphene and carbon nanotubes

Graphite, graphene and carbon nanotubes are all different forms of the element carbon. Graphene and carbon nanotubes are very useful as nanomaterials. The table on the next page summarises their different structures.

In each case, one electron per carbon atom is unbonded and delocalised, and is hence free to move and carry charge. Thus all three materials are electrical conductors.

> **Tip:** Remember that graphite, graphene and carbon nanotubes are all forms of the same element – carbon.

	Graphite	Graphene	Carbon nanotubes
Diagram of structure	Carbon atoms arranged in hexagonal layers. Covalent bond. Weak forces between layers.	Carbon atoms arranged in a single-atom-thick layer. Covalent bond.	Graphene sheet arranged in a cylinder.
Description of structure	**Layers** of carbon atoms are arranged in hexagons, with covalent bonds between the atoms and weak forces between the layers. This is a three-dimensional structure. Each carbon atom is covalently bonded to three others.	A **one-atom-thick sheet** of graphite with strong covalent bonds between each carbon atom. The atoms are arranged in hexagons. This is a two-dimensional structure. Each carbon atom is covalently bonded to three others.	A **one-atom-thick sheet** of graphene arranged in a **cylinder** with a hollow centre. This is a three-dimensional structure. Each carbon atom is covalently bonded to three others.

Physical properties of carbon nanotubes

Carbon nanotubes have useful physical properties. These include:

- high tensile strength and being very strong when pulled – this is due to the many strong covalent bonds throughout their structures;
- a high thermal and electrical conductance – because some of the electrons are delocalised and so can move and carry charge;
- being hollow – this means that a carbon nanotube can be used for delivery of drugs into specific parts of the body with the drugs carried inside the hollow centre of the molecule;
- an enhanced solubility; and
- a very high surface area to volume ratio.

Potential uses for carbon nanotubes in health care

Carbon nanotubes have found particular applications in health care. Some uses include:

Nitric oxide sensors

Sensors using carbon nanotubes embedded in a gel can be injected under the skin to monitor the level of nitric oxide in the bloodstream. The level of nitric oxide is important because it indicates inflammation in the body, and the sensors allow this to be measured to monitor inflammatory disease.

Scaffolding for tissue regeneration

A scaffold is a framework that holds cells or tissues together. Carbon nanotubes can be used to improve the healing process for broken bones by providing a scaffold that new bone material can grow around. This speeds up the growth of new bone tissue.

Glucose biosensors

At present, diabetes sufferers monitor their blood glucose levels by inserting a small needle into the skin or using glucose monitoring strips to which blood must be applied. These methods are invasive, painful and often inaccurate. Carbon nanotubes can be used in non-invasive glucose biosensors, which are highly sensitive due to the high electrical conductivity and large surface area of the nanotubes.

Bio-stress sensors

A carbon nanotube undergoes a change in electrical resistance when experiencing stress or strain. This means that it acts as a piezoelectric material. The change in current can be measured, hence providing a way to measure the stress. A bio-stress sensor of carbon nanotubes can be embedded within orthopaedic plates and screws in bone grafts. The sensor can determine the state of bone healing by measuring the effect of a load on the plate or screw in the bone. A healed bone will bear a large load, whereas an unhealed bone will transfer the load to the plate or screw causing a change in resistivity in the sensor. This allows doctors to accurately assess patient healing and quantify how much stress the affected area can tolerate. The sensor is able to communicate this information wirelessly.

Drug loading capacity
Drug loading capacity is the ability of the material to entrap a certain active drug. If the loading capacity of a given material is 30%, it means that 30% of each particle's weight is composed of the drug. Current drug delivery systems include polymers and liposomes. However, due to their hollow cylinder shape, carbon nanotubes have much higher drug loading capacities and have good cell penetration capacities. This gives them potential for use as drug deliverers.

Selective cancer cell destruction
Current cancer treatments can cause adverse side effects and generally result in normal cells, not just cancer cells, being killed. Single-walled carbon nanotubes can instead be used in drug delivery in cancer treatment. They are more effective than current treatments because they **enhance the solubility** of the drug and so move through the body easily. This allows for more efficient drug delivery and allows **tumour targeting**. This means that the carbon nanotubes can target specific cancer cells and, as a result, a lower dosage is needed. This reduces the side effects associated with conventional treatments. In addition, the carbon nanotubes target specific cancer cells, whereas current treatments also kill or remove normal cells.

Carbon nanotubes have a high drug loading capacity, good cell penetration, can target specific sites not harming healthy cells, and are unreactive. These are all properties that make them very useful in the treatment of cancer.

The benefits and risks of nanotechnology to society
Nanotechnology has developed rapidly in recent years, and new uses for nanoparticles are being researched and discovered daily. However, the benefits of the technology are not without risks. Some of the benefits and risks are as follows.

> **Tip:** If you are asked to evaluate the use of nanotechnology in society you need to mention some benefits and some risks.

Benefits of nanotechnology
- Selective cancer cell destruction using carbon nanotubes reduces the dose of cancer drug needed, so the side effects are reduced. The nanotubes only target cancer cells with no effect on healthy cells.
- Nanoparticles can remove pollutants and organic contaminants from soil and groundwater after environmental disasters. They are highly reactive because of their high surface area to volume ratio and so they target contaminants at a faster rate than larger particles.
- Nanotechnology can benefit the energy sector. Items such as batteries, fuel cells and solar cells can be built to be smaller and are more effective, so reducing energy consumption.
- In manufacturing, nanoparticles are used with precision to produce a wide range of products that are often stronger, more durable, and lighter than their conventional equivalents. Nanoparticles are used in products such as sun creams, cosmetics, sports equipment and aircraft wings.
- Micro robots made from nanomaterials (called nanobots) could be used in heart surgery on a miniature scale. Nanobots injected into the body could float through the circulatory system to detect problems and treat them (e.g. by detecting blood disease and killing infections). While surgeons can remove cancer cells on a micro level, a nanobot could ensure that all cells, even nanoscale ones, are removed.
- The military could develop nanomaterial disassemblers to attack physical structures or even biological organisms at the molecular level during warfare.

Risks of nanotechnology
- Recent studies on mice have shown that carbon nanotubes have caused mesothelioma (cancer of the lining of the lung). This is a similar adverse effect to that of asbestos.
- There is a risk of privacy invasion. Virtually undetectable surveillance devices could dramatically increase the potential for spying on governments, corporations and private citizens.
- Untraceable weapons made with nanotechnology could be smaller than an insect, yet have the intelligence of a

supercomputer. This could change the nature of warfare or terrorism.
- Inhaling airborne nanoparticles from manufactured materials may lead to pulmonary disease. Researchers have found that when rats breathed in nanoparticles, the particles settled in the brain and lungs, causing increased inflammation, stress and skin aging.
- In the future, nanobots will be able to function within an organism. For example, they could be programmed to replace damaged cells in the body. The risk of this is that, if they suffer some kind of mutation, self-replicating nanobots may develop and could disassemble and consume all living matter on Earth while building more of themselves. This is called the 'grey goo' scenario.
- Some nanoparticle products may have unintended consequences and unknown effects. For example, silver nanoparticles used in socks to reduce foot odour or in toothpaste to kill bacteria are flushed into the waste water stream and may cause environmental damage. They may also cause harm in the body.

Industrial considerations

A scientist must be able to carefully select a material with the properties that best meets the needs of the user. In industry, there are additional external considerations that will influence the choice of material for a particular situation. These factors include the following:

- **Price**: The material needs to be affordable. For example, in situations where a strong metal is needed, iron or titanium are both strong and hence would be suitable choices. However, iron is the more common choice as it is much less expensive. The selling price of a product needs to cover the cost of raw materials, manufacturing costs, packaging and distribution. Manufacturers must carefully weigh up these costs before choosing a material for a particular purpose.
- **Environmental considerations**: All materials affect the environment in terms of the pollution created, energy used and the manner of disposal of the product at the end of its life. Raw materials must often be extracted from natural resources (e.g. metal ores are extracted from the ground). This process may damage the environment and, once used, the natural resource cannot be replaced. As a result, it is advisable to use renewable resources where possible and to consider the use of renewable energy.
- **The quality of the item required**: Most products have a finite lifespan and eventually wear out and are disposed of. Designers have to consider how long a product is intended to last and whether it can be safely disposed of when it is no longer needed. Using better materials, for example stronger or more chemically resistant materials, extends product life. Nevertheless, using a higher-quality product often means that less material is used when compared to using several short-lived replacements of lesser quality. This is better for the environment. However, manufacturers need to consider that a longer life means that they will sell fewer replacement products and perhaps make less profit.
- **Demand and availability**: When manufacturing a product from a material, research must be carried out to ensure both that the material is readily available and that there is a demand for the product. A given material may be very suitable for a particular use, but may be difficult to acquire.
- **Regulations**: Most manufacturing processes produce various kinds of **waste** as a by-product. Sometimes these by-products contain toxic substances harmful to people or the environment and these may be controlled by laws and regulations. Correct disposal regulations must always be followed. Industrial manufacturers must also follow strict health and safety guidance when using chemicals and machinery.

Tip: Make sure you can evaluate the external factors that influence the choice of material for a particular situation.

Questions

1. What is a smart material? [2 marks]
2. Name three types of smart materials. [3 marks]
3. State the difference between a photochromatic and a thermochromatic material. [2 marks]
4. A particular wire can return to its original shape on warming. Name the type of smart material it is made of and describe one practical application of this smart material. [2 marks]
5. What is a quantum-tunnelling composite? [2 marks]
6. Describe one application of QTCs. [1 mark]
7. State two ways in which a piezoelectric material can work. [2 marks]
8. Name the element found in graphite and graphene. [1 mark]
9. Draw a labelled diagram to show the structure of graphite. [2 marks]
10. Compare the structures of graphene and a carbon nanotube. [3 marks]
11. Compare the structures of graphene and graphite. [3 marks]
12. Why are carbon nanotubes good conductors of electricity? [1 mark]
13. Describe the potential use of carbon nanotubes in a nitric oxide sensor. [3 marks]
14. State two advantages of carbon nanotube glucose biosensors over glucose monitoring strips. [2 marks]
15. Evaluate the use of carbon nanotubes in cancer treatment compared to current cancer treatments. [4 marks]
16. Describe the use of carbon nanotubes in bio-stress sensors in detecting bone healing. [3 marks]
17. State two risks and two benefits of nanotechnology to society. [4 marks]
18. Name three external factors that are considered when choosing a material to use in a particular situation. [3 marks]

5.8 SEMICONDUCTORS

Students should be able to:

5.8.1 demonstrate an understanding of how the electron configuration of silicon makes it an excellent semiconductor material;

5.8.2 describe briefly how n-type and p-type doping allow current flow in doped silicon; and

5.8.3 apply their knowledge of doping to briefly explain diode behaviour;

Silicon as a semiconductor

An atom's atomic number indicates the number of protons it contains and, because an atom is neutral in terms of electric charge, is also equal to the number of electrons in an atom. As described in section 5.2, in an atom, electrons are arranged in shells. The first shell holds two electrons, the next eight and the next eight. Silicon has an atomic number of 14. This means that silicon has 14 electrons and 14 protons. The electronic configuration (arrangement) of silicon can be written 2,8,4. The electronic configuration for silicon is shown in the diagram below, using a dot to represent each electron.

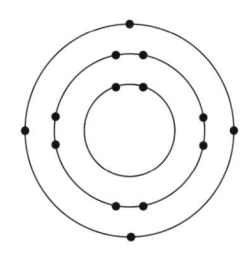

Electronic configuration for silicon

Elements that have **four outer shell electrons**, such as silicon and germanium, are excellent **semiconductors**. Semiconductors are materials that can conduct electricity under some conditions but not others.

In a crystal of pure silicon each silicon atom is bonded to four other silicon atoms, as shown in the next diagram. Pure silicon at room temperature is a poor conductor of electricity because all the outer shell electrons are bonded and so there are no delocalised electrons to move and carry the charge. However, pure silicon can be made to conduct electricity by the process of **doping**.

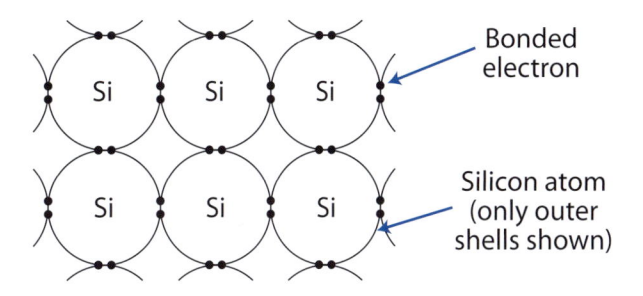

Crystalline structure of pure silicon at room temperature

Doping

Doping is the process of adding impurities to a semiconductor to change its electrical properties. Doping can be used to produce two different types of semiconductor, known as **n-type** and **p-type** semiconductors.

n-type semiconductors

Pure silicon can be changed into an n-type semiconductor by doping (adding) a small amount of an impurity element that has **five electrons** in the outer shell, such as phosphorus, arsenic or any Group V element.

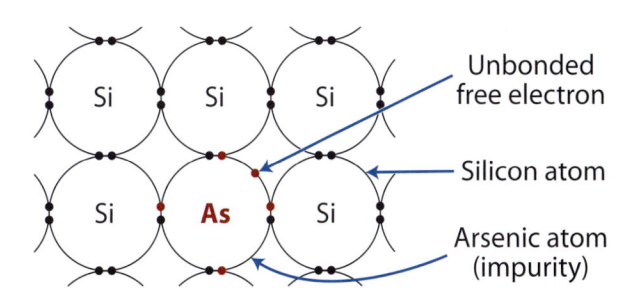

Crystalline structure of silicon with arsenic impurity added

The impurity atoms fit into the crystal structure by using four of their electrons to bond to other silicon atoms but, since these atoms have five electrons in the outer shell, one is left unbonded and can move and carry charge. Hence the impurity causes the material to become an electrical conductor. The majority charge carriers are negative electrons. The diagram above shows the crystalline structure of silicon with arsenic added to turn it into a n-type semiconductor.

> **Tip:** A charge carrier is a particle that is free to move and carry an electric charge. Examples are electrons and holes (see overleaf).

p-type semiconductors

Pure silicon can be changed into a p-type semiconductor by doping with a small amount of an impurity element that has **three electrons** in the outer shell. For example, a Group III element such as boron or aluminium can be added.

The impurity atoms fit into the crystalline structure by using their three outer shell electrons to bond to silicon atoms, but there is an electron missing. The area in the crystal where there is an electron missing is called a **positive hole**. An electron moves into the hole, creating a new hole nearby. By this process, the hole moves and so the current flows along the material from hole to hole. The majority charge carriers are positive holes. The diagram shows the crystalline structure of silicon with boron added to turn it into a p-type semiconductor.

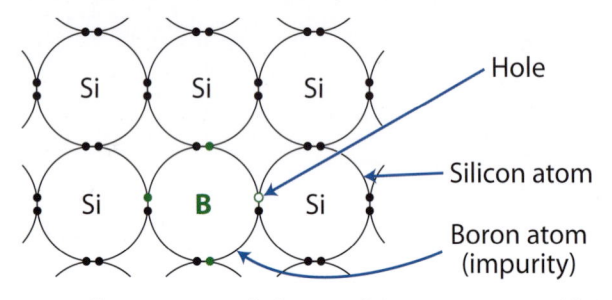

Crystalline structure of silicon with boron impurity added

Summary of n-type and p-type semiconductors

The table compares n-type and p-type silicon semiconductors.

	n-type semiconductor	p-type semiconductor
Impurity added	Elements with five electrons in outer shell, such as phosphorus or arsenic	Elements with three electrons in outer shell, such as boron or aluminium
Number of electrons present	Excess electrons	Deficiency of electrons
Majority charge carriers	Negative electrons	Positive holes

Diodes

Diodes are electrical components that allow current to flow in only one direction. They are built using semiconductor principles.

The circuit symbol for a diode is ⊹▷⊢−.

A p-n junction diode consists of n-type and p-type silicon **bonded** together. At the junction between the two materials, electrons from the n-type silicon fill in the holes in the p-type silicon. As a result, there are no charge carriers (neither free electrons nor positive holes) in this area and so it does not conduct electricity. The area is called the **depletion layer** as shown in the diagram below. The positive side of the diode is the p-type material. There are two ways to connect a diode, known as **reverse-biased** and **forward-biased**.

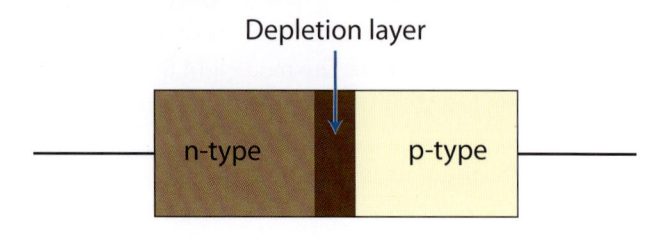

Arrangement of silicon in a p-n junction diode

Reverse-biased diode

To connect the diode in reverse-bias, the **n-type** material is connected to the **positive** terminal and the **p-type material** to the **negative** terminal of a battery, as shown in the diagram. The lamp in this circuit will not light.

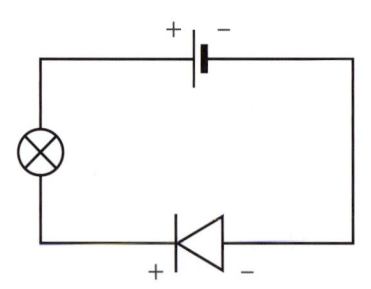

Circuit diagram containing a reverse-biased diode

Once connected, the negative terminal of the battery pulls positive holes from the p-type material away from the depletion layer and the positive terminal pulls electrons from the n-type material away from the depletion layer. This means that the depletion layer **increases in width** (i.e. gets bigger) so the diode does not conduct.

5.8 SEMICONDUCTORS

Bigger depletion layer

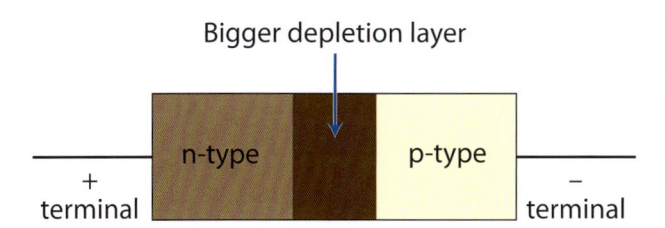

Arrangement of silicon in a p-n junction diode connected with reverse-bias

Tip: You may be asked to draw a circuit diagram showing a diode in reverse- or forward-bias. It is useful to include a bulb in your circuit, as it will indicate whether current is flowing.

Forward-biased diode

To connect the diode in forward-bias, the **n-type** material is connected to the **negative** terminal and the **p-type** material to the **positive** terminal of a battery, as shown in the diagram below. The lamp in this circuit will light.

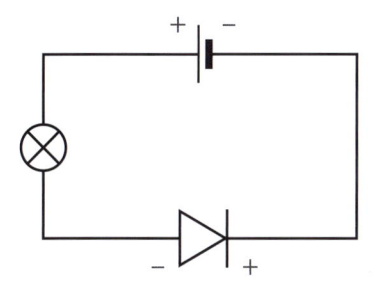

Circuit diagram containing a forward-biased diode

Once connected to the battery, the electrons and the holes both move into the depletion layer and fill it with charge carriers. This causes the depletion layer to **disappear** and the diode conducts. Diodes only allow electricity to pass when they are connected in the forward-bias manner. This means that diodes allow current to flow in only one direction.

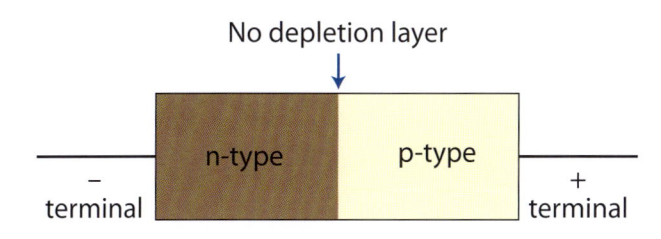

Arrangement of silicon in a p-n junction diode connected with forward-bias

Tip: To remember how to connect a diode in **forward-bias**, remember that **n** is connected to **n**egative and **p** to **p**ositive. For **reverse-bias** it is the **reverse** of this.

Questions

1. Silicon has atomic number 14. Write down its electronic configuration. [1 mark]
2. Explain why pure silicon is a poor conductor of electricity. [2 marks]
3. What is doping? [2 marks]
4. Name an element that can be added to silicon to make an n-type semiconductor, and explain how an n-type semiconductor conducts electricity. [3 marks]
5. Name an element that can be added to silicon to make a p-type semiconductor, and explain how a p-type semiconductor conducts electricity. [3 marks]
6. Name the majority charge carrier in a p-type semiconductor. [1 mark]
7. State three differences between n-type semiconductors and p-type semiconductors. [3 marks]
8. What is a diode? [1 mark]
9. How is a p-n junction diode built? [1 mark]
10. What is the depletion layer in a diode? [2 marks]
11. How is a diode connected in a circuit to achieve reverse-bias? [1 mark]
12. Draw a circuit diagram showing a battery in series with a lamp and a diode in forward-bias. [2 marks]
13. Explain why a diode conducts electricity when connected in forward-bias. [3 marks]

Answers

Note: The marks for each answer are for guidance only. Mark allocation may vary depending on the questions in the exam.

Unit AS 2: Human Body Systems

2.1 THE CARDIOVASCULAR SYSTEM

1. (a) Biconcave shape to increase surface area to volume ratio. [1]
   Absence of nucleus allows more space for haemoglobin. [1]
   (b) Passes into right ventricle and from there pumped through pulmonary artery to the lungs. [1]
   Blood becomes oxygenated in the lungs and there is a reduction in carbon dioxide content. [1]
   Passes through pulmonary vein to the left atrium. [1]
   Passes into left ventricle and from there is pumped at high pressure into the aorta. [1]
   [6 marks]

2. (a) Permeable/thin one-cell thick walls. [1]
   Formed of squamous endothelium. [1]
   Extensive network of capillaries provides a large surface area across which exchange can take place. [1]
   (b) Higher blood pressure closer to the heart (than in more distant arteries). [1]
   The increased amount of elastic tissue allows the arteries to expand more as the blood pulses through (at a greater pressure). [1]
   [5 marks]

3. (a) Any one from:
   The blood goes through the heart twice for each circuit of the body.
   There are two distinct circulations, the pulmonary (lung) and the systemic (body) circulations. [1]
   (b) The atrial walls contract [1]
   forcing blood into the ventricles. [1]
   (c) (i) The heart is beating too fast. [1]
   (ii) Any one from: palpitations / chest pain / dizziness / fainting / other appropriate response. [1]
   [5 marks]

4. (a) (i) 125 mm Hg [1]
   (ii) High blood pressure [1]
   (iii) Any one from:
   Damages blood vessels.
   Puts a strain on the heart (leading to a heart attack, stroke, organ damage). [1]
   (iv) The cuff is placed around the upper arm. [1]
   Cuff is inflated to reduce/stop blood flow down the arm. [1]
   Pressure is reduced to (initially) detect systolic pressure and (subsequently) diastolic pressure. [1]

(b) (i) Exercise [1]
(ii) Muscles [1]
require increased oxygen (and glucose) [1]
for the increased respiration required to produce energy (for the increased muscular activity). [1]

[10 marks]

2.2 RESPIRATORY SYSTEM

1. (a) Haemoglobin has four polypeptide chains each with an iron-rich haem group that can combine with oxygen. [1]
   Once one oxygen molecule has combined with haemoglobin, conformational change in the haemoglobin makes it easier for the other three molecules to combine. [1]
   (b) (i) The partial pressure of oxygen is the proportion of total air pressure that is contributed to by oxygen. [1]
   (ii) A physical change in haemoglobin in higher carbon dioxide levels/higher temperature/lower pH [1]
   that reduces its affinity for oxygen/causes it to release oxygen more readily [1]
   making more oxygen available to the tissues [1]
   allowing aerobic respiration to continue at times of greatest need (e.g. during strenuous exercise). [1]

   [7 marks]

2. (a) (External) intercostal muscles contract pulling the ribs up and out. [1]
   The diaphragm (muscle) contracts and flattens [1]
   increasing the volume and decreasing the pressure of the thorax (causing air to enter the lungs). [1]
   (b) (i) Ventilation/breathing bringing oxygen-rich air into the lungs. [1]
   Oxygen-rich blood in the lung capillaries is moved away. / Blood returning to the lungs is low in oxygen. [1]
   (ii) Surface area of gas exchange surface. [1]
   Thin and permeable exchange surfaces. [1]

   [7 marks]

3. (a) (i) In both men and women the PEF values increase and then decrease with age. [1]
   Men have a higher PEF value than women at all ages. [1]
   (ii) Muscle volume/strength of men increases to a peak in their 30s. [1]
   As they get older they have reduced muscle volume/strength. [1]
   (b) (i) Tidal volume is the amount of air normally breathed in and out during breathing. [1]
   Vital capacity is the maximum amount of air that can be breathed out following a maximum inhalation. [1]

(ii) They have reduced gas exchange due to damage to alveoli/exchange area. [1]
Higher breathing rate is to compensate (for the reduced exchange). [1]

[8 marks]

2.3 RESPIRATION

1. (a) Breathing is the process of taking air rich in oxygen and removing air rich in carbon dioxide to and from the lungs [1]
   to enable a high concentration gradient to be maintained for gas exchange. [1]
   Respiration is the process of breaking down glucose/carbohydrate to release energy [1]
   in body cells. [1]
   (b) The minimum amount of activity needed for the body to 'tick over' when completely at rest. [1]

   [5 marks]

2. (a) Adenine, ribose sugar and (three) phosphate groups. [1]
   (b) By one phosphate group/inorganic phosphate [1]
   joining to adenosine diphosphate (ADP). [1]

   [3 marks]

3. (a) (i) One [1]
   (ii) Hydrogen/electrons pass through a series of hydrogen/electron carriers in the electron transport chain. [1]
   At progressively lower energy levels / Series of redox (oxidation and reduction) reactions take place. [1]
   At certain points enough energy is released to synthesise ATP. [1]
   (iii) As there are two turns of the Krebs cycle during the respiration of each glucose molecule, this produces 4 CO_2. [1]
   Carbon dioxide is also produced in the link reaction. [1]
   Again, as two link reactions for each glucose molecule, 2 CO_2 are produced. [1]
   (b) Matrix [1]

   [8 marks]

4. (a) Two. [1]
   (b) Allows extra ATP to be produced above and beyond the maximum produced by aerobic respiration. [1]
   (c) Lactate. [1]

   [3 marks]

2.4 HOMEOSTATIC MECHANISMS AND HOW THESE ARE MONITORED

1. (a) (i) The maintenance of a constant internal environment/steady state. [1]
   (ii) Any two from: blood pH / blood glucose concentration / temperature / water potential / ion content / any other appropriate response. [2]
   (b) Any two from:
   Increases heart rate.
   Increases rate/depth of breathing.
   Raises blood glucose level.
   Causes blood vessels to contract to redirect blood toward major muscle groups, including the heart and lungs. [2]
   [5 marks]

2. (a) (i) β-cells (in islets of Langherans) [1]
   (ii) Any three from:
   Insulin lowers blood glucose concentration.
   Converts glucose to glycogen.
   Increases cellular respiration.
   Increases rate of glucose uptake into cells.
   Increases rate at which glucose is converted to fat. [3]
   (iii) Any three from:
   Glucagon increases blood glucose concentration.
   Stimulates liver cells to break down glycogen to glucose, releasing it into the blood.
   Speeds up the rate at which amino acids and other substances are converted to glucose.
   Reduces the rate of respiration. [3]
   [7 marks]

3. (a) (i) Any two from:
   Increases basal metabolic rate.
   Increases heart rate.
   Increases cardiac output.
   Increases ventilation rate.
   Potentiates/enhances the effects of the catecholamines (i.e. increases sympathetic activity).
   Potentiates/enhances brain development.
   Thickens endometrium/lining of utertus in females.
   Increases metabolism of proteins and carbohydrates.
   Promotes growth. [2]
   (ii) Pituitary (gland) [1]
   (b) (i) Increase [1] (ii) Decrease [1]
   [4 marks]

4. (a) (i) 94 to 99% [1]
   (ii) Using a pulse oximeter. [1]
   (iii) Due to breakdown of alveoli/reduced surface area/less gas exchange [1] breathing rate increases. [1]
   [4 marks]

2.5 NUTRITION AND PHYSICAL EXERCISE IN MAINTAINING GOOD HEALTH

1. (a) Any two from: milk / cheese / named dairy food / green leafy vegetables (e.g. broccoli, cabbage, and kale) / tofu / soya beans / sardines / white bread / any other appropriate response. [2]
   (b) Any two from: formation of bones and teeth / blood clotting / nerve function / muscle contraction / any other appropriate response. [2]
   (c) Vitamin D [1]
   [5 marks]

2. (a) Energy intake from food exceeds energy expended by the body. [1]
   Extra energy is stored by the body as fat. [1]
   Body mass is gained. [1]
   (b) (i) Helps the release of energy from carbohydrates/fats/proteins. [1]
   Required for functioning/maintenance of nerves. [1]
   (ii) Any two from: fortified breakfast cereals / wholegrain breads / liver / potatoes / peas / eggs / any other appropriate response. [2]
   (iii) Beri beri [1]
   [8 marks]

3. (a) Any two from: oily fish / liver / milk / eggs. [2]
   (b) Any one from: rickets / osteomalacia [1]
   (c) No direct sunlight in winter months. [1]
   Lack of vitamin D made by the body. [1]
   Vitamin D aids in absorption of calcium/phosphate. [1]
   Strong bones/bone development of baby described. [1]
   [7 marks]

4. (a) (i) Spread units evenly over three or more days. [1]
   Reduce units to 14 units per week / man is consuming 2 units more than recommended. [1]
   (ii) Any two from:
   High blood pressure.
   Stroke.
   Liver disease.
   Different types of cancer.
   Mental health problems, including depression.
   Damage to the brain and nervous system.
   Pancreatitis.
   Sexual problems, such as impotence. [2]
   (b) (i) Protein is lower/10 g lower than recommended. [1]
   Vitamin C is lower/15 mg lower than recommended. [1]
   Protein source – any one from: beans / pulses / fish / eggs / meat / any other appropriate response. [1]
   Vitamin C source – any one from: Fruit / vegetables / citrus fruits (e.g. oranges, lemons and limes) / green or red peppers / tomatoes / broccoli / potatoes / any other appropriate response. [1]
   (ii) $\frac{5}{9} \times 100$ [1] = 55.56% [1]
   [10 marks]

ANSWERS

Unit AS 3: Aspects of Physical Chemistry in Industrial Processes

3.1 CHEMICAL CALCULATIONS

1. (a) 58.5 [1] (b) 17 [1] (c) 213 [1] (d) 331 [1]
   (e) 74 [1] (f) 164 [1] (g) 400 [1] (h) 98 [1]
   [8 marks]

2. (a) $\frac{16}{58}$ [1] = 0.28 [1]   (b) $\frac{50}{100}$ [1] = 0.50 [1]
   (b) $\frac{54}{342}$ [1] = 0.16 [1]   (d) $\frac{5.6}{74}$ [1] = 0.076 [1]
   [8 marks]

3. (a) 0.3 × 40 [1] = 12 g [1]
   (b) 0.25 × 74 [1] = 18.5 g [1]
   (c) 1.2 × 106 [1] = 127.2 g [1]   [6 marks]

4. In each of (a) – (c), award [1] for conversion to g [1] for relative formula mass and [1] for final answer.
   (a) mol = $2.1 \times \frac{10^6}{160}$ = 13125 [3]
   (b) mol = $\frac{1220}{148}$ = 8.24 [3]
   (c) mol = $\frac{3200}{100}$ = 32 [3]   [9 marks]

5. (a) 0.25 × 3 = 0.75 [1] (b) $\frac{1.2}{3}$ = 0.4 [1]   [2 marks]

6. (a) 84 [1]   (b) $\frac{2.1}{84}$ = 0.025 [1]
   (c) $2NaHCO_3 : 1Na_2CO_3$
       0.025 : 0.0125 [1]
   (d) mass = 0.0125 × 106 [1] = 1.325 g [1]   [5 marks]

7. moles $Pb(NO_3)_2$ = $\frac{33.1}{331}$ = 0.1 mol [1]
   ratio: 2 : 4
                1 : 2
                0.1 : 0.2 [1]
   mass = 0.2 × 46 = 9.2 g [1]   [3 marks]

8. moles = $\frac{mass}{M_r}$ = $\frac{475000}{95}$ [1] = 5000 [1]
   ratio: $1MgCl_2 : 2HCl$
       5000 : 5000 × 2 = 10000 [1]
   mass of HCl = moles × M_r = 10000 × 36.5
               = 365000 g [1]
               = 365 kg [1]   [5 marks]

9. mol of NH_3 = $\frac{6200}{17}$ [1] = 364.7 [1]
   mol of NO = 364.7 [1]
   mass of NO = 364.7 × 30 = 10941 g theoretical [1]

   % = $\frac{8000}{10941}$ × 100 [1] = 73.1% to 1 d.p. [1]   [6 marks]

10. (a) $\frac{23.5}{94}$ = 0.25 [1]
    0.25 : 0.25 [1]
    0.25 × 197.5 = 49.4 g [1]
    (b) $\frac{38.1}{49.4}$ [1] × 100 = 77.1% = 77% [1]   [5 marks]

3.2 VOLUMETRIC ANALYSIS

1. (a) mol = $\frac{120}{40}$ = 3 mol in 2 dm³ [1]
   $\frac{3}{2}$ = 1.5 mol dm⁻³ [1]
   (b) mol = $\frac{3.4}{17}$ = 0.2 mol in 200 cm³ [1]
   0.2 × 5 = 1 mol dm⁻³ [1]
   (c) mol = $\frac{5.3}{106}$ = 0.05 mol in 250 cm³ [1]
   0.05 × 4 = 0.2 mol dm⁻³ [1]   [6 marks]

2. (a) 4 × 0.3 = 1.2 [1] (b) 1.5 × 2.0 = 3.0 [1]
   (c) $\frac{100 \times 1.5}{1000}$ = 0.15 [1] (d) $\frac{25 \times 0.5}{1000}$ = 0.0125 [1]
   [4 marks]

3. (a) A solution of known concentration. [1]
   (b) Strong alkali/strong acid [1] so use methyl orange (red to yellow) or phenolphthalein (colourless to pink). [1] for named indicator [2] for correct colour change.   [5 marks]

4. (a) 1.8 g in 250 cm³ is 7.2 g in 1 dm³ [1]
   $\frac{7.2}{40}$ = 0.18 mol dm⁻³ [1]
   (b) Weigh out 1.8 g of NaOH in a clean dry beaker using a top pan balance. [1]
   Dissolve the solid in a small volume (50–100 cm³) of deionised water. Stir with a glass rod. [1]
   Transfer the solution to a 250 cm³ volumetric flask. [1]
   Rinse the beaker and glass rod with deionised water and add the rinsings into the volumetric flask. [1]
   Make up to the mark by adding deionised water until the bottom of the meniscus is on the mark. [1]
   Stopper the flask and invert to mix thoroughly. [1]
   [8 marks]

5. (a) moles of NaOH = $\frac{16.4 \times 0.400}{1000}$ = 0.00656 [1]
   $\frac{0.00656}{2}$ = 0.00328 [1]
   $\frac{0.00328 \times 1000}{20.0}$ = 0.164 mol dm⁻³ [1]
   (b) It is a strong acid, strong alkali titration. [1]
   [4 marks]

6. (a) moles of HCl = $19.8 \times \dfrac{0.0500}{1000} = 0.00099$ [1]
   (b) ratio 2 HCl + Ca(OH)$_2$
       $\dfrac{0.00099}{2} = 0.000495$ [1]
   (c) $\dfrac{0.000495 \times 1000}{25.0} = 0.0198$ mol dm^{-3} [1]

   [3 marks]

7. (a) Rinse the pipette with the barium hydroxide solution. [1]
       Use a safety pipette filler and draw up the solution until the bottom of meniscus is on the line. [1]
       Release the solution from the pipette into a conical flask. [1]
       Touch the pipette on the surface of the liquid to remove the last drops in the pipette. [1]
   (b) Any eight from [* **must be included**]:
       Rinse the burette with deionised water, then hydrochloric acid and discard the rinsings.
       Fill the burette with hydrochloric acid.
       Make sure the jet is filled and there are no air bubbles in the burette.
       Record the volume at the bottom of the meniscus at eye level to 1–2 decimal places (if two decimal places are used, the second decimal place must be 0 or 5.).
       * Add 2–3 drops of phenolphthalein or methyl orange to the conical flask.
       Add the acid from the burette, swirling the conical flask.
       Continue addition until the indicator just changes from pink to colourless/yellow to pink.
       The volume should be recorded, reading to the bottom of the meniscus at eye level.
       Repeat the titration but add the solution dropwise near the end point. Record the volume added.
       Repeat the titration until the results are concordant (within 0.1 cm^3 of each other).
       Calculate the mean of the accurate titrations. [8]
   (c) (i) 22.3 and 22.4 [1]
       (ii) Use the two accurate titres to calculate the mean:
            $\dfrac{22.3 + 22.4}{2} = 22.4$ cm^3 [1]
       (iii) moles = $\dfrac{22.4 \times 0.200}{1000} = 0.00448$ [1]
       (iv) Ba(OH)$_2$: 2HCl
            $\dfrac{0.00448}{2} = 0.00224$ [1]
       (v) $\dfrac{0.00224 \times 1000}{25.0} = 0.0896$ mol dm^{-3} [1]

   [17 marks]

8. (a) moles of HCl = $\dfrac{12.4 \times 0.100}{1000} = 0.00124$ [1]
   (b) $\dfrac{0.00124}{2} = 0.00062$ [1]
   (c) $\dfrac{0.00062 \times 1000}{25.0} = 0.0248$ mol dm^{-3} [1] **[3 marks]**

3.3 ENERGETICS

1. Any two from:
   In an exothermic reaction, heat is given out; in an endothermic reaction, heat is taken in.
   In an exothermic reaction, the temperature of the surroundings increases; in an endothermic reaction, the temperature of the surroundings decreases.
   Exothermic reaction energy change value is negative; endothermic energy change value is positive. [2]

   [2 marks]

2. 298 K (25°C) [1], a pressure of 100 kPa. [1] **[2 marks]**

3. The energy taken in to break bonds in carbon dioxide and water [1] is greater [1] than the energy given out when bonds are made in glucose and oxygen. [1]

   [3 marks]

4. The activation energy (E_a) is the minimum energy needed for a reaction to occur. [1] **[1 mark]**

5. Reaction profile similar to below with the following labelled: axes [1], energy change [1], activation energy [1] and products below reactants [1].

   [4 marks]

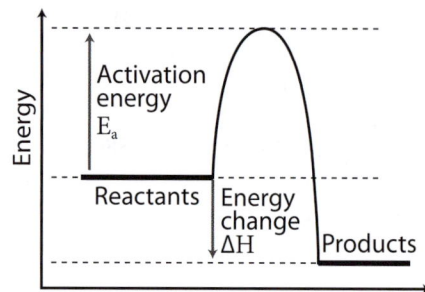

6. (a) Average bond enthalpy is the energy required to break one mole of a given bond [1] averaged over many compounds. [1]
   (b) Bonds broken = $348 + (5 \times 412) + 264 + 463 + (3 \times 496) = 4623$ [1]
       bonds made = $(4 \times 803) + (6 \times 463) = 5990$ [1]
       enthalpy change = $4623 - 5990 = -1367$ kJ mol^{-1} [1]
   (c) Bond energies are average values. [1]
   (d) Enthalpy change of combustion is the enthalpy change when 1 mole of a substance [1] is completely burnt in oxygen (under standard conditions). [1]
   (e) Any eight points from:
       Measure a volume of water (e.g. 100 cm^3) into a calorimeter/beaker using a measuring cylinder.
       Weigh a spirit burner containing the liquid fuel to be burnt.
       Measure the initial temperature of water using a thermometer (T_1).
       Place the spirit burner under the calorimeter and light the wick.
       When there is a reasonable temperature rise (15°C), stop heating and extinguish the flame.

Stir and measure the final temperature (T_2) of the water using a thermometer.
Cool and reweigh the spirit burner.
Calculate temperature change (ΔT) = $T_2 - T_1$ and the heat energy change in joules using $Q = mc\Delta T$.
Calculate the mass of fuel used in the burner by subtraction, and calculate the number of moles of fuel used.
Calculate the energy change per mole of fuel used. [8]
[16 marks]

7. 436 + 242 – 2H–Cl = –186 [2]
   2H–Cl = 864 [1]
   H–Cl = 432 kJ mol^{-1} [1] **[4 marks]**

8. (a) moles = $\dfrac{1.54}{88}$ [1] = 0.0175 [1]
   (b) ΔH = 180 × 4.18 × (75.3–22.8) [1] = –39501 J for 0.0175 moles [1]
   2257200 J mol^{-1} [1] = –2260 kJ mol^{-1} (3 s.f.) [1]
   [note the value is negative because heat is given out]
   (c) Any two from: incomplete combustion / non-standard conditions / evaporation of water / heat loss to surroundings. [2]
   (d) 366 + (5 × –394) + (6 × –286) = –3320 kJ mol^{-1} [3]
   [11 marks]

9. ΔH = 277 + (–394 × 2) + (–286 × 3)
   = 277 – 788 – 858
   = –1369 kJ mol^{-1} **[3 marks]**

10. ΔH = (–394 × 4) + (–286 × 5) + 2880
    = –1576 – 1430 + 2880
    = –126 kJ mol^{-1} **[3 marks]**

3.4 KINETICS

1. (a) The rate of a reaction is a measure of the speed at which reactants are changed into products. [1]
   (b) Activation energy (E_A) is the minimum energy needed for a reaction to occur. [1]
   [2 marks]

2. The 2.0 mol dm^{-3} acid has higher concentration, so there are more particles present in the same volume [1] and more successful collisions in a given time. [1]
   [2 marks]

3. Powder will react faster as there is a greater surface area, so more particles on the surface exposed to the acid [1] and more successful collisions in a given time. [1] **[2 marks]**

4. (a) (i) D [1] (ii) C [1] (iii) A [1]
   (b) An exothermic reaction [1] as products have less energy than reactants. [1] **[5 marks]**

5. (a) A catalyst is a substance that increases the rate of a reaction [1] without being used up. [1]
   (b) It provides a different pathway of lower activation energy [1], so more particles have greater energy than the activation energy [1] and more successful collisions in a given time. [1]
   (c) The catalyst is solid and in a different state [1] from the gaseous reactants. [1]
   (d) It bonds to the active site [1] and stops the catalyst from working. [1]
   (e) It increases surface area to speed up the reaction. [1]
   (f) Reactants are adsorbed on to the surface of the catalyst [1], causing bonds to weaken in the reactant molecules and products to form. [1] Product molecules desorb and leave the active site available. [1]
   (g) (i) iron [1] (ii) platinum-rhodium [1] **[15 marks]**

6. (a) When the temperature is increased, particles gain energy and move faster. [1] A higher proportion of the particles will possess more energy than the activation energy [1], so there are more successful collisions in a given time. [1]
   (b) peak is lower [1], peak moves right. [1]
   [5 marks]

7. (a) Stopclock / flask connected to gas syringe / measuring cylinder or pipette to measure volume of acid / balance to weigh calcium carbonate. [3] for listing 4 pieces, [2] for 3 pieces, [1] for 2 pieces of apparatus.
   (b) Any two from: use same volume of acid / use same mass of carbonate / use same particle size of carbonate / use same concentration of acid. [2]
   (c) Steeper for higher temperature [1] but finishes at same time. [1]
   (d) When the temperature is decreased, particles lose energy and move slower. [1] A smaller proportion of the particles will possess more energy than the activation energy [1], so there are fewer successful collisions in a given time [1].
   [10 marks]

3.5 EQUILIBRIUM

1. (a) A reversible reaction is one in which the products, once made, can react to reform the reactants. [1]
   (b) Dynamic equilibrium occurs in a closed system [1] when the rates of forward and reverse reactions are equal and the amounts of reactants and products remain constant. [1] **[3 marks]**

2.

	Haber process	Contact process
Symbol equation	$N_2 + 3H_2 \rightleftharpoons 2NH_3$ [2]	$2SO_2 + O_2 \rightleftharpoons 2SO_3$ [2]
Temperature (°C)	450°C [1]	450°C [1]
Pressure (atm)	200 atm [1]	1–2 atm [1]
Catalyst	Iron [1]	vanadium (V) oxide [1]

[10 marks]

3. (a) Pressure – the position of equilibrium moves to the right [1] as there are fewer molecules on the right. [1]
   (b) Temperature – the position of equilibrium moves to the left [1] in the endothermic direction (to remove heat). [1] **[4 marks]**

4. (a) High pressure – the right-hand side has fewer molecules [1] and increased pressure causes equilibrium position to move right, giving a higher yield. [1]
   (b) High pressure is expensive. [1]
   (c) Low temperature – reaction is exothermic [1] so a lower temperature causes equilibrium to move right, giving a higher yield. [1]
   (d) Low temperature means a slow rate. [1] **[6 marks]**

5. (a) It is an exothermic reaction [1] so increasing the temperature causes the equilibrium position to move left in the endothermic direction. [1]
   (b) Increasing the pressure causes the equilibrium position to move to the left [1], as there are fewer molecules (3½) compared to 4 molecules on the right. [1] **[4 marks]**

6. A closed system. [1] **[1 mark]**

3.6 INDUSTRIAL PROCESSES

1. (a) The cost of setting up a business or plant [1], e.g. any one from: construction of manufacturing plant / plant equipment / storage for raw materials / design fees. [1]
   (b) Direct – e.g. any two from: crude oil / fuel / transport of raw material or product. [2]
       Indirect – e.g. any two from: insurance / rent / sales / maintenance / labour. [2]
   (c) A non-stop process where products are removed as reactants are added. [1]
   (d) An intermittent process where reactants are added, a reaction occurs and products are removed. The vessel is cleaned and the process is started again. [1]
   (e) (Generally) faster / less labour intensive. [1]
   (f) An unprocessed material from which a product is made. [1] **[10 marks]**

2. Any three from: eyesore / noise pollution / acid rain / destruction of natural habitats / water pollution / thermal pollution / air pollution. [3] **[3 marks]**

3. (a) Indirect [1] (b) Capital [1] (c) Direct [1]
   (d) Indirect [1] (e) Direct [1] **[5 marks]**

Unit AS 5: Material Science

5.1 MATERIAL PROPERTIES

1. Density = $\frac{mass}{volume}$ = $\frac{500}{8.1 \times 6.0 \times 5.0}$ [1] = 2.1 g cm^{-3} [1] **[2 marks]**

2. Density = $\frac{mass}{volume}$ = $\frac{1.30}{0.36 \times 0.55 \times 0.0025}$ [1]
   = 2.6×10^3 kg m^{-3} [1] = 2.6×10^6 g m^{-3} [1] **[3 marks]**

3. $9.0 \times 10^3 \times 0.00050$ [1] = 4.5 kg [1] **[2 marks]**

4. $2400 \times 1.5 \times 2.0 \times 3.0$ [1] = 2.2×10^4 kg (2 s.f.) [1] **[2 marks]**

5. Density = $\frac{mass}{volume}$; so $1.07 = \frac{mass}{250}$ [1]
   giving mass = $1.07 \times 250 = 267.5$ g [1]
   For water: $1.00 = \frac{mass}{250}$, giving mass = 250 g of water [1]
   mass of sodium chloride = 267.5 − 250 = 17.5 g [1] **[4 marks]**

6. (a) Thermal conductivity is a measure of the ability of a material to conduct heat. [1]
   (b) Electrical conductivity is a measure of the ability of a material to carry an electrical current. [1]
   (c) Chemical resistance is the strength of a material to withstand chemical attack. [1] **[3 marks]**

7. (a) a metal (e.g. copper) [1]
   (b) air / any gas [1] **[2 marks]**

8. B. [1]
   As it reacted less vigorously with the acid. [1] **[2 marks]**

9. Electrical conductivity = $\frac{L}{RA}$ = $\frac{0.25}{6.0 \times 10^{-8} \times 4.2}$ [1]
   = 992063.49 = 9.9×10^5 [1] S m^{-1} [1] **[3 marks]**

10. Micrometer [1] **[1 mark]**

11. (a) A = $\frac{\pi d^2}{4}$ [1]
    (b) Cross section area bigger by × 4 [1] **[2 marks]**

12. (a) Diamond [1] in the form of a square-based pyramid [1] with 136° between faces [1] is used to indent the material.
    (b) Between 10 N and 1000 N / between 1g and 100g [1] for a time of 10–15 s. [1]
    (c) Vickers hardness number (VHN) / N m^{-2}. [1] **[6 marks]**

ANSWERS

13. **(a)** Stress (σ) is the applied force per unit cross section area. [1] Strain (ε) is the extension (change in length) per unit length. [1]
    Young modulus (E) = $\frac{\text{stress }(\sigma)}{\text{strain }(\varepsilon)}$,
    i.e. the ratio of stress and strain. [1]
    (b) Initial length of wire: metre stick. [1]
    Diameter of wire: micrometer screw gauge. [1]
    Extension of wire: Vernier arrangement / metre stick. [1]
    Masses: use a balance and multiply by *g* or use a newton meter. [1]
    (c) So that the extension is large enough to read. [1]
    [8 marks]

14. The extension ΔL = 190 − 160 mm = 30 mm [1]
    $\varepsilon = \frac{\Delta L}{L_O} = \frac{30}{160} = 0.1875$ [1]
    $E = \frac{\sigma}{\varepsilon}$, so σ = Eε = 2.0×10⁷ × 0.1875
    = 3.75×10⁶ N m⁻² [1]
    F = σA = 3.75×10⁶ × 0.64×10⁻⁶ = 2.4 N [1]
    [4 marks]

15. $\sigma = \frac{F}{A} = \frac{80}{1.3\times10^{-6}} = 6.15\times10^7$ N m⁻² [1]
    $E = \frac{\sigma}{\varepsilon}$, so 2.0×10¹¹ × ε = σ [1]
    So 2.0×10¹¹ × ε = 6.15×10⁷
    giving ε = 6.15×10⁷ ÷ 2.0×10¹¹ = 3.075×10⁻⁴ [1]
    $\varepsilon = \frac{\Delta L}{L_O}$ [1], so ΔL = ε × L_O = 3.075×10⁻⁴ × 150
    So ΔL = 4.6×10⁻² m [1]
    [5 marks]

16. **(a)** A: limit of proportionality [1] B: elastic limit [1]
    C: yield point [1] D: breaking point [1]
    (b) Wire E [1]: it has the higher gradient. [1]
    (c) Wire G [1]: it stretches elastically and breaks, with no plastic deformation. [1]
    [8 marks]

5.2–5.3 CATEGORISING MATERIALS AND MICROSCOPIC STRUCTURE

1. **(a) (i)** protons and neutrons. [1]
   (ii) electrons in shells/energy levels. [1]
   (iii) protons in the nucleus. [1]
   (b) According to the Bohr model, there is an equal number of protons and electrons in the atom, so their charges cancel out. [1] **[4 marks]**

2. Delocalised electrons [1] can move and carry charge. [1]
   [2 marks]

3. Layers of ions can slide over each other [1], yet the delocalised electrons still attract the ions and hold the structure together. [1] **[2 marks]**

4. Crystalline, as their structure has a regular or ordered arrangement of particles. [1]
   [1 mark]

5. A large molecule made of many repeated units called monomers [1] joined in a long chain molecule. [1]
   [2 marks]

6. A thermoplastic can be heated and reshaped [1] many times as there are only weak forces between the polymer chains and these are easily broken. [1] Thermosets can only be heated and shaped once [1] as they have strong crosslinks between the chains. [1]
   [4 marks]

7. **(a)** There are weak intermolecular forces [1] between polymer chains and these forces are easy to break. [1]
   (b) There are cross links/strong bonds between the polymer molecules [1] and these bonds take a lot of energy to break. [1]
   [4 marks]

8. Composites combine different materials [1] to create a material with better, more useful, properties than any of its components. [1]
   [2 marks]

5.4–5.5 ALLOYS, METAL WORKING AND BIOMATERIALS

1. It is a mixture of two or more elements [1] (copper and zinc) and at least one of the elements is a metal. [1]
   [2 marks]

2. Iron [1] and nickel. [1]
   [2 marks]

3. Any three from:
   Both contain iron.
   There is a greater percentage of iron in steel.
   Steel contains mainly iron and carbon, with small amounts of chromium, manganese and vanadium.
   Stainless steel contains mainly iron and chromium with small amounts of carbon, nickel and manganese. [3]
   [3 marks]

4. Copper [1] and tin. [1]
   [2 marks]

5. Any two from: Musical instruments / door locks / door bolts [2].
   [2 marks]

6. Any two from: thermostats / clock mechanisms / watch mechanisms. [2]
   [2 marks]

7. Annealing is the process of heating a metal [1] to a temperature above its recrystallization temperature [1] and then letting it cool slowly. [1]

[3 marks]

8. To make a metal softer / easier to cut / easier to work [1].

[1 mark]

9. Any two from: stainless steel heart stents / titanium pacemakers / synthetic skin / metal hip or knee joints / bioglass implants. [2]

[2 marks]

10. Bioinert: does not release toxins, is not rejected by the body and does not react with biological tissue [1]. However, a bioactive material does react with adjacent biological tissues in the body. [1]

[2 marks]

11. Bioactive – because it bonds directly with the biological tissue. [1]

[1 mark]

12. Any two from: strong / corrosion resistant / biotolerant. [2]

[2 marks]

13. Any one from: titanium / stainless steel. [1]

[1 mark]

14. A biomaterial is one that is inserted into the body as part of a medical device. [1]

[1 mark]

5.6, 5.7, 5.9 SMART MATERIALS, NANOMATERIALS AND INDUSTRIAL CONSIDERATIONS

1. Smart materials have physical properties that change [1] in response to an external condition such as temperature, light, pressure or electricity. [1]

[2 marks]

2. Any three from: shape-memory alloys / piezoelectric materials / quantum-tunneling composites / thermochromatic materials / photochromic materials / electroluminescent materials. [3]

[3 marks]

3. Thermochromatic materials change colour in response to a change in temperature. [1] Photochromatic materials change colour reversibly in response to a change in light. [1]

[2 marks]

4. Shape-memory alloy [1]. Practical application, any one of: spectacle frames if bent and heated return to normal shape / holding bones in place / cold nitinol stents can be inserted into a blood vessel where they then expand at body temperature to the correct diameter, to keep the vessel open / dental braces. [1]

[2 marks]

5. This material is a flexible polymer that contains tiny metal particles. [1] It is an insulator but if it is squeezed it becomes a conductor. [1]

[2 marks]

6. Any one of: touch switches / touchscreens / motor speed controllers / pressure sensors. [1]

[1 mark]

7. When put under stress (e.g. when a mechanical force is used to bend or change their shape by squeezing, a piezoelectric material produces a voltage). [1] When a voltage is applied to a piezoelectric material the material changes shape. [1]

[2 marks]

8. Carbon. [1]

[1 mark]

9. See diagram on page 119. Labels must be included and at least 2 layers. [2]

[2 marks]

10. Both are a one-atom-thick sheet of graphite. [1] Both have carbon atoms arranged in hexagons with each carbon bonded to 3 others. [1] Both have one electron per carbon atom unbonded and delocalised. [1] Graphene is a two-dimensional sheet, carbon nanotubes are three-dimensional hollow cylinders. [1]

[4 marks]

11. Graphite is in layers; graphene is a one-atom-thick sheet. [1] Both have carbon atoms arranged in hexagons, with each carbon atom bonded to 3 others. [1] Both have one electron per carbon delocalised. [1]

[3 marks]

12. Delocalised electrons [1] can move and carry charge. [1]

[2 marks]

13. Carbon nanotubes embedded in a gel can be injected under the skin as sensors [1] to monitor the level of nitric oxide in the bloodstream. [1] Nitric oxide indicates inflammation in the body, allowing monitoring of inflammatory disease. [1]

[3 marks]

14. Any two from: non-invasive / painless / accurate. [2]

[2 marks]

15. Any four from: Current cancer treatments cause adverse side effects and all normal cells are killed. [1] Carbon nanotubes enhance solubility and so move through the body easily. [1] This allows for more efficient drug delivery [1] and so a lower dose is needed, causing fewer side effects. [1] Carbon

nanotubes can target specific cancer cells and don't harm normal cells. [1]

[4 marks]

16. Any three from: A bio-stress sensor of carbon nanotubes is placed in orthopaedic plates and screws in bone grafts. [1] A load is applied to the sensor. [1] A healed bone will bear a large load; however an unhealed bone transfers the load to the plate or screw causing a change in current [1] in the sensor which is measured wirelessly. [1]

[3 marks]

17. Any two risks [2] and any two benefits [2] from the lists on pages 120 and 121.

[4 marks]

18. Any three from: price / environmental considerations / quality required / demand and availability / regulations [3].

[3 marks]

5.8 SEMICONDUCTORS

1. 2,8,4 [1]

[1 mark]

2. All four outer shell electrons of silicon are bonded to other silicon atoms [1] and so there are no delocalised electrons to move and carry the charge. [1]

[2 marks]

3. Doping is the process of adding impurities [1] to a semiconductor to change its electrical properties. [1]

[2 marks]

4. Any Group V element (e.g. phosphorus, arsenic). [1] The impurity has five electrons in the outer shell and four are used to bond to silicon atoms [1], leaving one over to move and carry charge. [1]

[3 marks]

5. Any Group III element (e.g. boron, aluminium). [1] The impurity uses three outer shell electrons to bond to silicon atoms [1], but there is an electron missing, forming a positive hole. Electrons move into the holes and so the current flows along the material from hole to hole. [1]

[3 marks]

6. Positive hole. [1]

[1 mark]

7. In n-type, the majority charge carriers are negative electrons, in p-type, they are positive holes. [1] Those of n-type have an excess of electrons, while p-type have a deficiency of electrons. [1] In p-type, a group III element is used to dope, in n-type a group V element is used. [1]

[3 marks]

8. Diodes are components that allow current to flow in only one direction. [1]

[1 mark]

9. A p-n junction diode is built by bonding n-type silicon and p-type silicon together. [1]

[1 mark]

10. The area at the junction of a diode where electrons from the n-type silicon fill in the holes in the p-type silicon [1] and, as a result, there are no charge carriers and no conduction in this area. [1]

[2 marks]

11. To connect the diode in reverse-bias, the n-type material is connected to the positive terminal and the p-type material to negative material. [1]

[1 mark]

12. [2]

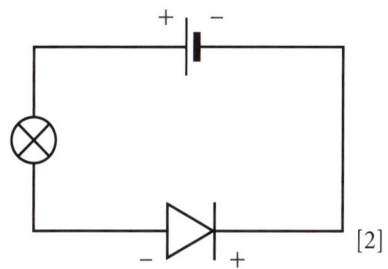

[2 marks]

13. The electrons and the holes both move to the depletion layer [1] and fill it with charge carriers. [1] This causes the depletion layer to disappear and the diode conducts. [1]

[3 marks]